I0101992

Secret CBD Cures For Seniors

The Natural Healing Breakthrough for Pain Free Longevity

Brooke Tilson, MSG

with Kristina Etter

Copyright © 2020 by Brooke Tilson

All rights reserved.

No part of this book may be reproduced in any form or by any electronic or mechanical means, including information storage and retrieval systems, without written permission from the author, except for the use of brief quotations in a book review.

Secret Cures Publishing, LLC

ISBN: 978-1-952208-00-3

Interior Design: Kristen Forbes of DeviancePress.com

Praise for *Secret CBD Cures for Seniors*

"*Brooke Tilson has written the definitive guide to CBD for Seniors. Whether for chronic pain, insomnia or mood swings, thousands are finding relief from the aches and pain that often accompany the aging process. Secret CBD Cures for Seniors is timely and offers insights into the rapidly changing cannabis landscape. Brooke provides answers to questions you might not have thought to ask.*"

– **Dexter Rusell**, MD

"*If you want to wake up refreshed for an early-morning walk, or help reduce anxiety or ease joint pain, and are considering using CBD, check out this book.*"

– **Kathy Smith**, Fitness, Longevity, & Wellness Legend

"*Pain in our body is something we all confront as we age, and is often too big to handle on our own. CBD offers a natural alternative to pain killers that have adverse or addictive side effects.*"

– **Kyra Wong**, Accredited Exercise Therapist
& CEO of Pain Free Studio

"As our population ages, it is important to continually educate and inform our Seniors about Natural and plant-based options to both promote well-being and prevent disease. This book does a great job introducing this key demographic to Cannabidiol, a popular compound derived from Cannabis known as CBD, and much more."

– Robert "Doc Rob" Streisfeld, NMD

"Given the increased scrutiny of the traditional medications that we use for pain management including opioids, nonsteroidal anti-inflammatory medications and neuropathic medications the side effect profile for each of these is significant and real. This is why I have been advocating for CBD use in the health care providers pain management armamentarium. This is especially important for our senior population where drug interactions and polypharmacy play a large part in medication related dangers. I believe CBD is a real and promising alternative that can provide real pain relief for this specific patient population."

– Jerome Julian Grove, MD

"I highly recommend this natural oil to anyone who suffers from chronic pain, anxiety or sleep disorders. Thank you Brooke Tilson for

providing such important healing information!"

                – **Lauren Lockey**, Health & Wellness Expert

"All natural CBD holds incredible potential…. Especially for Seniors!"

                – **Lisa S. Abrams**, MD

This book is dedicated to everyone, regardless of age, that gets up each morning with total conviction that the best days of their lives are still to come. These optimistic warriors choose faith over fear and have the courage to explore new paths that can lead their lives in positive new directions.

DISCLAIMER

The contents of this book are provided for general informational purposes only, and in no way should be construed as medical advice. The information presented here is not meant as a substitute for, or alternative to, information from professional health care practitioners. CBD products are not intended to diagnose, treat, cure or prevent any disease. Please consult your health care professional before initiating any new nutritional supplementation to review potential interactions or other possible complications that could arise from using any new product. The authors, publishers, and distributors of this book do not endorse any medical claims or anecdotal stories presented in this book. The statements made regarding CBD products, and the efficacy of these products, have not been evaluated by the Food and Drug Administration. The author and the publisher do not accept responsibility, nor shall be held liable, for any adverse effects individuals may claim to experience, whether directly or indirectly, from information contained in this book.

CONTENTS

Part 3 | Getting Started With CBD

FOREWORD

The emerging field of cannabinoid medicine offers us exciting possibilities for health and wellness. At its forefront is cannabidiol (CBD).

Although CBD was initially discovered 80 years ago, it has only received heightened attention by medical research in the last decade. Since that time, understanding of its therapeutic benefits has been exponential in growth. Presently, peer-reviewed clinical research as well as subjective patient testimony indicate that cannabidiol has a role in multiple disease states, including those related to inflammation, pain, mental health and potentially even cancer.

As a board-certified physician and neuroscientist investigating the therapeutic benefits of CBD, I have witnessed first-hand its success in the treatment of patients with autoimmune disease, anxiety, insomnia, chronic pain and addiction.

With the alarming prevalence of polypharmacy within the aging population and its associated health risks, widespread interest in CBD therapeutics could not arrive at a better time.

Fortunately there are those with a passion for demystifying the science of cannabinoid medicine and currently known medicinal benefits of CBD. Brooke Tilson is one such individual, and thoughtfully achieves this in her book.

Relying on her undergraduate and graduate training at the USC Leonard Davis School of Gerontology, she successfully distills cannabinoid research and communicates CBD's therapeutic benefits in clear and concise language. I hope, as does Brooke, that by reading this book you will gain a practical understanding of CBD and how it can promote health and wellness in the aging population.

Christian Shaw, MD PhD

www.rebelmd.com

PREFACE

CBD is everywhere these days. Unfortunately, the people that can benefit the most from CBD—Seniors—are unaware of the most recent scientific advancements and health research on this miraculous natural medicine.

This book is going to change all that.

You're about to discover an entire universe of CBD products available to you now, and how they can help you enjoy a new, restful life… free from stress, pain, and anxiety.

The 5 Most Important Things You Need to Know About CBD

We all know the time-proven life lesson: "if you can protect yourself on the downside, the upside will take care of itself." Here are five critical facts that should alleviate many of your concerns as you explore the benefits of CBD:

1. **CBD is all-natural.**
2. **CBD is safe and non-addictive.**
3. **CBD is super affordable.**
4. **CBD is legal.**
5. **CBD won't get you high.**

With these common concerns taken care of, let's talk about the possible mind-blowing medical benefits of introducing CBD supplementation into your life.

Imagine Saying Goodbye to Your Chronic Pain Conditions!

This is not a misprint. Many people from every walk of life are reporting that CBD can significantly reduce, and in some cases, totally eliminate the following chronic pain issues:

- **Inflammatory Pain**
- **Many types of Arthritis**
- **Osteoarthritis**
- **Spinal Stenosis**
- **Degenerative Disc Disease**
- **Gout**
- **Plantar Fasciitis**
- **Migraines**

Lift the Cloud of Stress, Anxiety, and Other Mental Health Disorders Affecting Your Life!

Mental health conditions can be challenging to treat effectively. Research is starting to show that CBD may help people seeking a solution for the following ailments:

- **Anxiety**
- **Depression**
- **Schizophrenia**

- **PTSD**
- **Mood Disorders**
- **Stress**

Get Help Now for the Devastating Effects of Your Autoimmune Disorders!

Make no mistake about it. CBD may very well be your best solution for successfully fighting the frustrating symptoms of a plethora of autoimmune disorders including:

- **Addison's Disease**
- **Celiac Disease**
- **Chronic Fatigue Syndrome**
- **Fibromyalgia**
- **Grave's Disease**

- **Hashimoto's Disease**
- **Psoriasis**
- **Lupus**

Diminish the Symptoms of Neurological Diseases that Threaten Your Quality of Life!

It's no secret that neurological diseases can negatively change the trajectory of our lives in a multitude of horrific ways. CBD supplementation has proven to be effective in protecting the brain and significantly reducing symptoms associated with:

- Huntington's Disease
- Parkinson's Disease
- Multiple Sclerosis
- Alzheimer's Disease
- Stroke
- ALS
- Epilepsy
- Dementia

But that's not all!

CBD also has a wide range of antioxidant benefits and cardio-protective properties. **Additionally, CBD can help mitigate some of the unpleasant side effects of cancer treatments as well as promote healthy, restorative sleep.**

Does this Make CBD a Miracle Cure?

Despite all the incredible possible benefits outlined above, I would discourage you from rushing to the conclusion that CBD is a fast and easy solution for all of your medical conditions.

But what I will encourage you to do, is mindfully explore how CBD can best benefit YOU, so you can start living the life of your dreams, that you so rightfully deserve. **You have everything to gain, and absolutely nothing to lose!**

PART 1

CBD & SENIORS: GET READY FOR THE BEST YEARS OF YOUR LIFE

1

CBD: A NEW MEDICINE FOR A NEW YOU

"Disease has a way of getting you down to the point where you just give up and get used to it. If there is anything working with CBD oil has shown me, it's that there is always hope. Even for the hopeless."

— **Michael J. Fox, Actor**

Aging is an unavoidable fact of life. Yet, in modern American society, getting older is dreaded, feared, and even treated like another chronic disease we're supposed to mitigate at all costs.

Why are we brainwashed into fearing our futures? Unfortunately, because big business has discovered it's quite profitable to tell us this is the case.

Here's the situation...

Due to advances in fitness, nutrition, and technology, life expectancy has reached unprecedented levels. By 2035, there will be more people over the age of 65 than children under the age of 18.[1] **This makes Seniors a ridiculously lucrative target market for every business in the world.**

This has motivated every C Suite executive in today's largest corporations to become laser-focused on creating new products and services that are geared to fulfill the needs of this vast and newly emerging segment of our population.

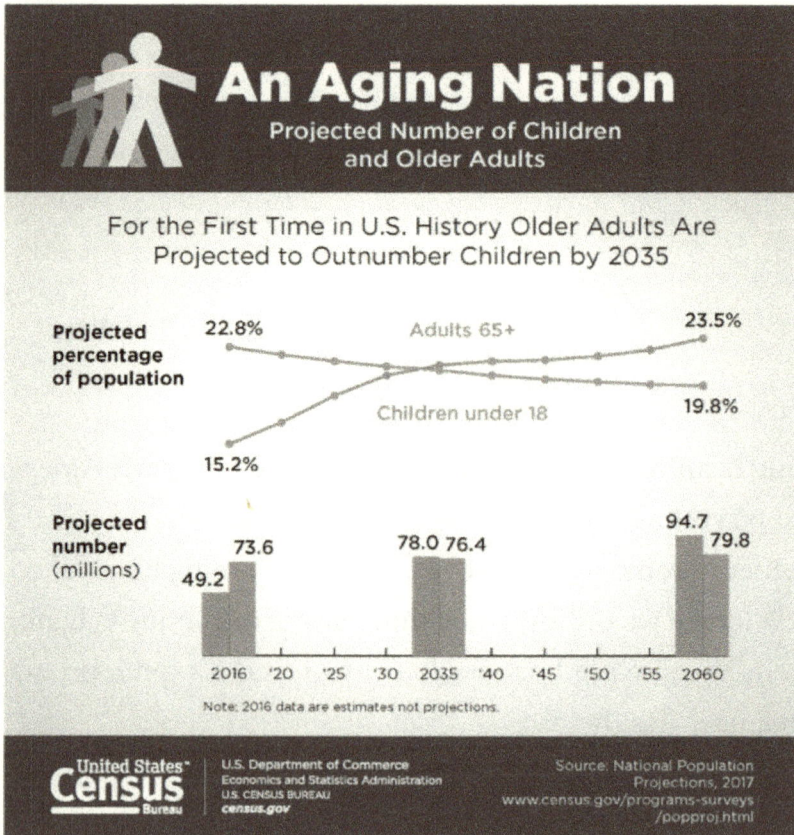

An Aging Nation
Projected Number of Children and Older Adults

For the First Time in U.S. History Older Adults Are Projected to Outnumber Children by 2035

Projected percentage of population

Adults 65+ 22.8% ... 23.5%
Children under 18 15.2% ... 19.8%

Projected number (millions)

| 2016 | '20 | '25 | '30 | 2035 | '40 | '45 | '50 | '55 | 2060 |

49.2 73.6   78.0 76.4   94.7 79.8

Note: 2016 data are estimates not projections.

United States Census Bureau

U.S. Department of Commerce
Economics and Statistics Administration
U.S. CENSUS BUREAU
census.gov

Source: National Population Projections, 2017
www.census.gov/programs-surveys/popproj.html

As legendary aging expert, Ashton Applewhite reminded during her, "Let's End Ageism" lecture on TED,[2]

> *"Who says wrinkles are ugly? The multi-billion-dollar skin care industry. Who says perimenopause and low-T and mild cognitive impairment are medical conditions? The trillion-dollar pharmaceutical industry."*

Our fear of aging starts early. As children, we're taught to believe that aging is a sad fact of life. Movies and television depict Seniors as frail, weak, sick, and lonely.

Based on these stereotypes, we create negative mental images of how we should look and act, and pessimistic expectations about our quality of life. This results in us fighting the aging process, as we try to maintain our younger selves and deny the inevitable.

This fear of aging is unproductive, extremely destructive, and a terrible waste of time and energy.

So, remember this: No matter what anyone tells you, old age isn't something you need to fix. **Growing older is part of the natural progression of life, which you should celebrate and embrace, not fear and reject.**

Applewhite also tells us,

"It's embarrassing to be called out as older until we quit being embarrassed about it… it's not healthy to go through life dreading our futures."

Learning how to accept and embrace the aging process starts with reinventing our idea of what getting older means and represents. Even though our society widely reinforces ageism, I'm here to tell you that aging comes with benefits:

- **With age, we acquire wisdom.**
- **With age, we learn patience.**
- **With age, we learn to accept our flaws.**
- **With age, our empathy and social skills improve.**
- **With age, we have more time to enjoy life.**

Best of all, with age, it appears we also maintain a greater sense of happiness.

Your Happiest Days are Scientifically Proven to be Ahead of You

Interestingly, researchers have long been aware there is a mental and emotional phenomenon that comes with age. Regardless of nationality, race, sex, or religion, everyone shares a similar pattern in terms of measuring happiness throughout life. This pattern is universally recognized as the U-Curve of Happiness.

As it turns out, we are the happiest at the beginning and the end of our lives. While people often compare the ebb and flow of life's experiences with the ups and downs of a roller coaster, the U-Curve of Happiness shows, emotionally speaking, this comparison is accurate.

U-Curve of Happiness

Average life satisfaction by age
(Adjusted world sample, 2010–2012)

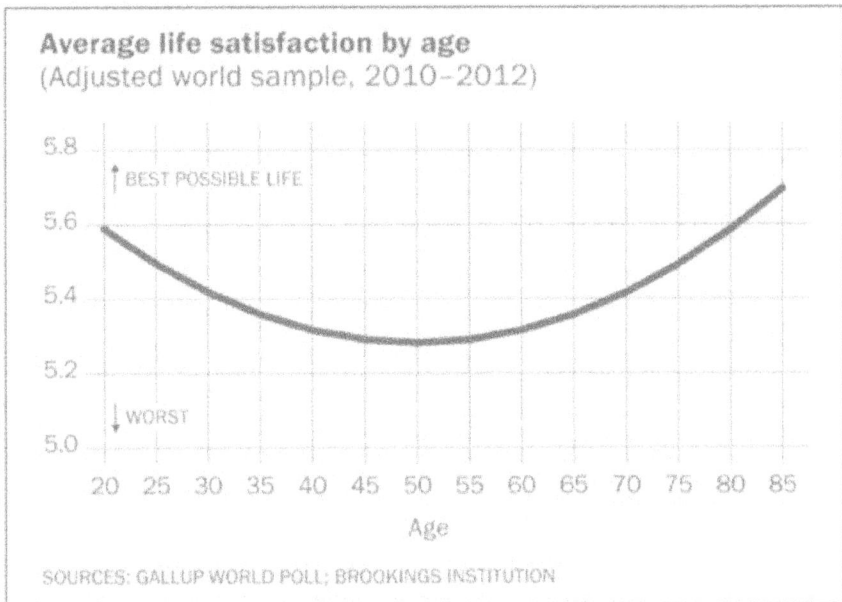

SOURCES: GALLUP WORLD POLL; BROOKINGS INSTITUTION

In his book, *Better With Age: The Psychology of Successful Aging*, Alan D. Castel from the University of California, believes that, in many ways, **life before 50 is really more of a training regimen – one which teaches us the art of aging and how to successfully become an older human being.**

While other books about aging speak about the process like

it's something to be avoided or prevented, Castel's book showcases new research which highlights critical paradoxes regarding how we think about aging versus how we age.

According to Castel's research, when we start blaming our flaws, our shortcomings, and our failures on "getting old," it is reinforced in our brains as a valid excuse for our decline in functionality.

You Deserve More from Life After 50!

When we complain about our aches and pains after the age of 50, we tend to say, "I'm just getting old." Yet, when we are younger, we would never carelessly accept these flaws as the status quo.

Likewise, when we misplace our car keys or TV remote after 50, it's quickly swept under the rug as a "Senior moment." This would never be a valid excuse for a lapse in memory when we are younger.

Castel suggests there may be a different way to approach the way we look at aging by centering our focus on the positives of growing old and realigning how we define them.

> *"It is not true that people stop pursuing dreams because they grow old; they grow old because they stop pursuing dreams."*
>
> – Gabriel García Márquez, Novelist

CBD: A New Medicine For a New You

If you're like most people, you are probably searching for life hacks that will allow you to live a longer, better, more active, and fulfilling life.

That's why it's so valuable to understand what CBD is, how it works, and the incredible benefits that this 100% all-natural modern medicine can offer you RIGHT NOW!

2

WHAT EXACTLY IS CBD?

"You don't have to take CBD, but you should at least know about it if it's going to help you protect your body."

— Derrick Morgan, NFL Player

Cannabidiol –or CBD– is one of many active, chemical compounds found in hemp and marijuana plants, which are called phytocannabinoids.

While the molecular structure of CBD is the same regardless of whether it is extracted from hemp or marijuana, the CBD we are discussing is derived from hemp, which means it contains less than .3% THC. **This means that hemp derived CBD is non-psychoactive and will not get you high.**

CBD attaches to receptors in our endocannabinoid system

to keep all our mental and physical processes running smoothly. The discovery of the endocannabinoid system is universally recognized as one of the most important medical breakthroughs of the past 50 years and will be fully explained later in this book.

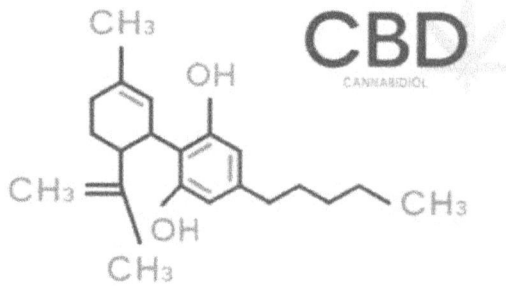

How CBD Oils are Made

When hemp plants have reached full maturity, they are ready for processing.

Extraction technicians grind up the plant material, or biomass, and use a solvent to pull the beneficial oils from the plant matter. This crude oil, which is often dark brown, green, or even black, is then refined using high-tech, lab equipment to remove residual solvents, waxes, and solids — leaving behind a golden, honey looking oil.

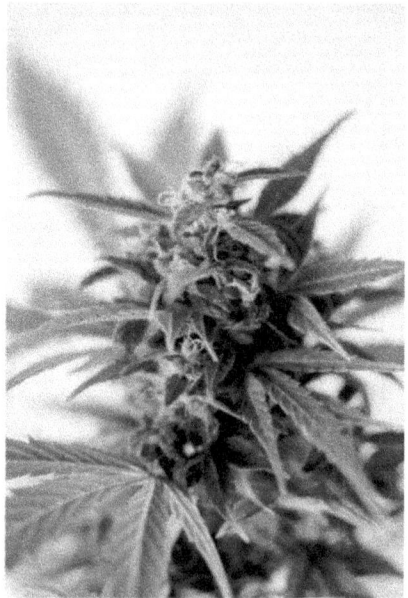

Some CBD manufacturers continue to refine the oil further. Using a process called chromatography, lab technicians can separate the crude oil into its individual components, including a spectrum of cannabinoids, terpenes, and other volatile substances. Many manufacturers are using this kind of extraction technology today to remove THC from oils entirely or to make CBD isolate powders.

Once the CBD oil is extracted from the hemp plant, it can be directly ingested and enjoyed in an endless array of product forms, including cookies, candies, drinks, and capsules. CBD can also be applied topically through balms, lotions, serums, cosmetics, and bath products.

3

11 REASONS WHY CBD IS A MIRACLE MEDICINE

"CBD helps with pain, stress and anxiety. It has all the benefits of marijuana without the high."

— Jennifer Aniston, Actor

Now that we know what CBD is, and where it comes from, let's examine the 11 main reasons why millions of people consider CBD to be a miracle medicine.

1. CBD is all-natural.

As explained in the previous chapter, CBD is extracted from hemp plants. It's an all-natural alternative to the expensive, man-made pharmaceuticals that are so brazenly dumped on

Seniors.

2. CBD is legal.

With the recent signing of the Farm Act Bill in December 2018, the United States declared that it is entirely legal to own hemp-derived CBD. As of this writing, just three States— Idaho, Nebraska, and South Dakota—fail to recognize the Farm Act Bill and say owning CBD is illegal.

3. CBD is very safe and non-addictive.

Clinical trials show that CBD has a very strong safety profile, which is non-habit-forming, safe for all ages, and has few side effects. Unlike many expensive, man-made pharmaceutical drugs, CBD won't cause physical addiction.

4. CBD is non-psychoactive – it won't get you high.

THC, which is found in marijuana, is well-known for its euphoric effects. Hemp-derived CBD contains less than .3% THC, which means it won't get you high or impair you in any way.

> *"I like CBD oil. There's no THC in it. You don't get high."*
>
> – Roger Daltrey, Musician

5. CBD is super affordable.

It's common to read headlines about the price gouging happening in the pharmaceutical industry. For example, people with diabetes are forced to ration their insulin, and people have died because they couldn't afford to replace their life-saving Epi-pen.

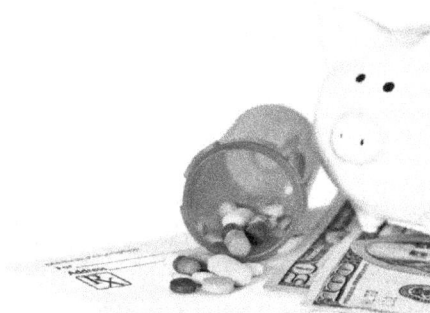

Now that hemp cultivation is completely legal, the supply of CBD has grown exponentially, and prices have fallen dramatically. CBD, in any form, is super affordable compared to the cost of many prescription medications on the market.

6. CBD acts as a pain reliever.

CBD is exceptionally effective at battling neuropathic pain, such as fibromyalgia and Multiple Sclerosis. **A survey completed by Brightfield Group showed that 42 percent of those using CBD reported reducing, if not quitting, their use of painkillers.**[3]

7. CBD is an effective anti-inflammatory.

CBD combats inflammation by exerting an immunosuppressive effect on specific cells that play a role in inflammation and immunity.[4] Research also shows CBD may reduce inflammatory pain by activating glycine receptors.[5]

> *"Rather than relying on potentially damaging anti-inflammatories like Tylenol and Advil, I have been turning to CBD and seeing incredible results without side effects."*
>
> — Sergio Pettis, MMA Athlete

8. CBD is a powerful antioxidant.

Similar to vitamins C and E, CBD can help reduce the damage done by oxidative stressors such as toxins, smoke, and pesticides.[6]

9. CBD is a potent anxiolytic.

Although CBD doesn't create an intoxicating effect, it certainly can assist those with mood disorders such as anxiety and depression.[7] **Freedom from stress and anxiety is one of the most popular reasons people explore CBD supplementation.**

10. CBD has neuroprotectant qualities.

Research has shown that CBD may help with central nervous system injuries such as spinal cord injury and disease, traumatic brain injury, and strokes. Additionally, CBD may also help slow down the progression of disorders like ALS, MS, epilepsy, and Parkinson's disease.[8]

11. CBD is a proactive medicine.

I'm sure you've heard the statement, "We don't have a health care system; we have a sick care system." The truth is, for decades, Western medicine has only included reactive treatments. Instead of preventing illness and disease before they occur, we rely on physicians and pharmaceuticals to make us better after we become sick. On the other hand, **CBD is a proactive, preventative medicine, helping to promote overall wellness and natural healing processes.**

❖

While CBD is grabbing the majority of headlines, there are dozens of other cannabinoids found in hemp, called minor cannabinoids, which hold a few secrets of their own.

4

MORE MIRACLES!
MINOR CANNABINOIDS, TERPENES,
AND FLAVONOIDS

"It's CBD. It helps with the healing process and inflamma-tion... It will make your life better."

— **Nate Diaz, MMA Athlete**

While CBD is the most abundant cannabinoid found in the hemp plant, **there are many other wonderfully healthy compounds included in top quality, full spectrum, and broad spectrum, CBD products.**

Also called whole-plant extractions, full spectrum CBD products contain all of the original compounds in the hemp plant: cannabinoids, terpenes, flavonoids, and even trace amounts of THC that by law cannot exceed 0.3% (meaning it won't get you high). These compounds are as close to the natural chemical makeup of the original plant as possible.

Researchers have found that when all of these compounds are combined together, they work to produce even more significant medical benefits than any single molecule does on its own. **Researchers have labeled this phenomenon of the sum of the whole hemp plant being greater than the parts, "The Entourage Effect."** Let's explore these exciting compounds and their therapeutic potential.

Minor Cannabinoids May Change Your Life in Major Ways

Over one hundred active compounds are found in the hemp plant. The therapeutic value of these compounds is just starting to be understood. With hemp cultivation recently legalized in the United States, we can look forward to exciting new research from major universities and research facilities. In the meantime, let's talk about what we know so far.

Here are the three minor cannabinoids we know the most about and their therapeutic benefits.

Cannabigerol – CBG

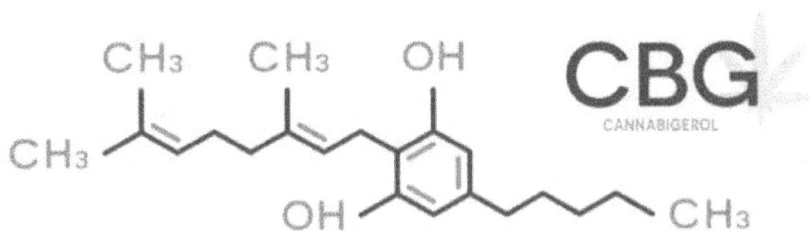

CBG, or cannabigerol, is referred to as the "Mother Cannabinoid" because it gives birth to CBD as the hemp plant matures. As such, producers and researchers often harvest plants early when they want to extract high quantities of CBG. Here's what a few early studies say about the benefits of CBG:

1. CBG slows down cancer growth.

Multiple studies have been conducted on the anti-cancer abilities of cannabinoids. Researchers published a study in 2006 that says CBG may work against breast cancer.[9] More recently, in 2016, another study stated that cannabinoids such as CBG could directly inhibit cancer tumor progression.[10]

2. CBG has antibacterial & antifungal properties.

Research published in 2008 in the Journal of Natural Products suggests CBG may be capable of fighting drug-resistant bacterial infections such as MRSA.[11]

3. CBG efficiently reduces inflammation.

Multiple studies indicate CBG may be better at controlling inflammation than even CBD. A study published in May of 2011 suggests CBG works exceptionally well for reducing cells responsible for inflammation.[12] Likewise, a study performed in 2013 showed CBG reduced colon inflammation in rats,[13] which suggests patients with inflammatory bowel disease may find some relief from CBG as well.

4. CBG is an extremely active neuroprotectant.

CBG could potentially help with neurodegenerative diseases such as Huntington's disease and Parkinson's disease. A study from 2015 showed CBG increased antioxidant defenses and worked exceptionally well as a neuroprotectant.[14]

5. CBG may help with anxiety and depression.

Dr. Ethan Russo published a review of cannabinoids in 2016, referring to CBG as the "neglected phytocannabinoid." Russo's report states that CBG has shown antidepressant capabilities in mice.[15] Additionally, Doctor Bonni Goldstein says that CBG also works as a GABA reuptake inhibitor, that produces calming, muscle relaxing, and anti-anxiolytic properties as well.[16]

Perhaps the most compelling evidence for the therapeutic potential of CBG comes from GW Pharmaceuticals, the company that is responsible for producing Epidiolex, the pharmaceutical-grade CBD medication that has received approval from the FDA. GW Pharmaceuticals filed for a patent on CBG for the treatment of around 50 different ailments and diseases including pain, neurodegenerative disease, brain injury, inflammatory and autoimmune diseases.[17]

Cannabinol – CBN

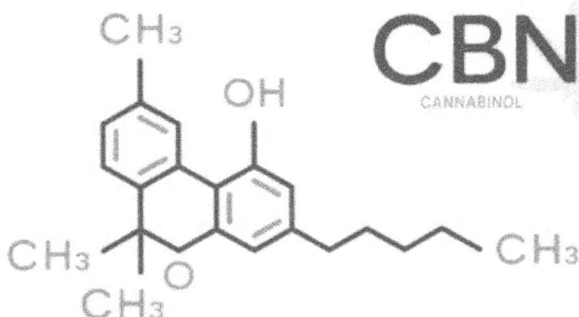

Just as CBG is the precursor to CBD, cannabinol, or CBN, is formed at the opposite end of the cannabinoid life cycle. **The inherent sleep-inducing qualities of CBN may hold promise for millions of Americans battling sleep disorders.**

Israel based Kanabo Research released a 2019 study showing multiple combinations, or formulas, of phytocannabinoids and how they help to fight insomnia and sleep disorders. Their research measured sleep duration of various cannabinoid formulations, and a combination of CBD, THC, and CBN revealed the best results.[18]

In fact, Steep Hill Labs, a highly respected cannabis research facility in California, also believes CBN is a valuable tool in the battle against sleeplessness. **Their website states CBN is almost twice as sedative as Valium.**[19]

Cannabichromene – CBC

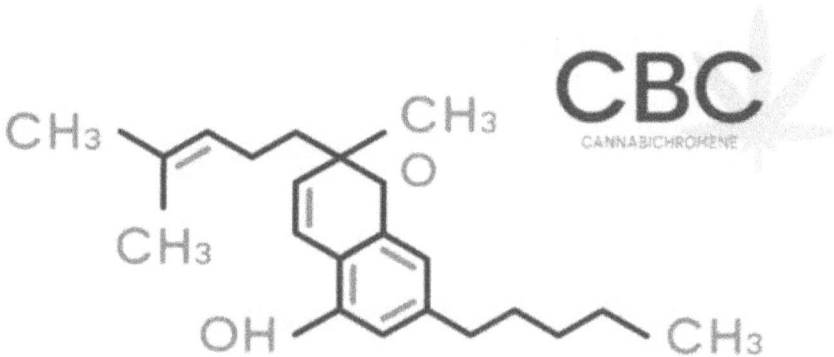

Cannabichromene (CBC) is actually the second most abundant cannabinoid found in the hemp plant. Structurally similar to CBD, the compound degrades into CBL (cannabicyclol) and CBT (cannabicitran), two other cannabinoids of interest to researchers.

Researchers are excited that CBC may have various medicinal applications, including:

- Anti-inflammation
- Nerve Pain Reduction
- Pain Relief
- Neuroprotection
- Antibacterial
- Antifungal

Additionally, many researchers believe CBC may be effective at reducing migraines, gastrointestinal disorders, and even acne.[20]

Terrific Terpenes Trigger Natural Healing

The terpenes included in full spectrum CBD also deliver tremendous health benefits. Although the term "terpenes" may be new to you, it's reasonable to assume that you consume terpenes each and every day without even realizing it. Terpenes are the molecules found in plants, herbs, and spices, which give them aroma and flavor.

For example, if you've ever sliced into a lemon and smelled the fresh citrus of the lemon rind, then you've consumed terpenes. If you put black pepper on your meals, you've consumed terpenes. If you've ever used a lotion or essential oil with natural lavender, then you've consumed terpenes. Let's explore the terrific terpenes found in the hemp plant and how they can benefit your health.

- **Limonene** – As the name implies, you encounter this terpene every time you slice a lemon. That sweet, citrusy aroma you inhale is limonene. Also found in citrus, juniper, and peppermint, **limonene may assist with gastric reflux, gallstones, and cancer.**[21]

- **Pinene** – This common terpene should conjure memories of Christmas, as pinene is what gives pine trees their familiar aromas. Also found in sage and rosemary, **pinene is used as an antiseptic, anti-inflammatory,**[22] **and as a natural bronchodilator for patients with breathing issues**. Pinene may also be useful in improving memory function and has been used as an anti-cancer treatment in Chinese Medicine.[23]

- **Myrcene** – Known to be relaxing, calming, and mildly sedating, myrcene can also be found in mangos and cloves. Dr. Ethan Russo's highly publicized 2016 research on CBD shows that **myrcene is a potent pain reliever, anti-inflammatory, and antibiotic,** and may also improve the functionality of other cannabinoids and compounds.

- **Caryophyllene** – Commonly found in spices such as black pepper, oregano, and basil, **this terpene has been studied for pain relief, anxiety reduction, inflammation relief, and as an antibacterial.**[24]

- **Humulene** – Also found in coriander and hops, this terpene is **considered anti-inflammatory, antibacterial, and pain-relieving.** Research from 2007 shows that combining **humulene with caryophyllene may produce vigorous anti-cancer activity as well.**[25]

- **Linalool** – Maybe one of the most common terpenes, linalool, is found in hundreds of plants and spices such as lavender, rosewood, mint, and cinnamon. Mildly sedating and extremely calming, **linalool is often used to help with sleep.** Research suggests linalool may be useful as an antibacterial, antifungal, and powerful antioxidant.[26]

Fierce Flavonoids Fight Inflammation

Other compounds found in hemp plants and full spectrum CBD are called flavonoids, which are also starting to gain massive attention for their potential, awe-inspiring therapeutic benefits.

There are 20 flavonoids commonly found in hemp. Of these, two of them, Cannflavin A and Cannflavin B, occur nowhere else in nature. **Recent research shows some flavonoids found in hemp may be up to 30 times more effective at treating inflammation than aspirin.**[27]

5

WHAT YOUR DOCTOR DIDN'T LEARN IN MEDICAL SCHOOL: THE ENDOCANNABINOID SYSTEM

"I have been a believer in the benefits of CBD for some time."

— John Legend, Musician

Most of us remember our high school anatomy lessons and learning about the major systems of the human body.

- **The Cardiovascular System** includes the heart, arteries, and veins which supply our body with blood.

- **The Respiratory System** consists of our lungs, which take in oxygen and expel carbon dioxide.

- **The Nervous System** is made up of the brain, spinal cord, and nerves.

- **The Digestive System** is our intestines and stomach.

- **The Immune System** protects us from diseases.

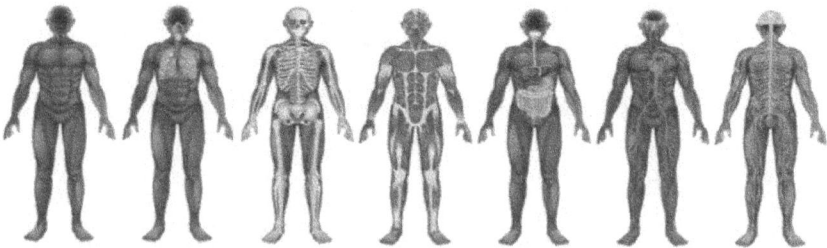

The Endocannabinoid System (ECS): The Most Significant Medical Finding of Our Time

During the late 1980s and early 1990s, a team of researchers, led by Dr. Raphael Mechoulam, uncovered an entire microscopic system woven into our cells, which they aptly named the Endocannabinoid System.

This major medical discovery is so recent that only 9 percent[28] of medical schools in the United States include it in their curriculum today.

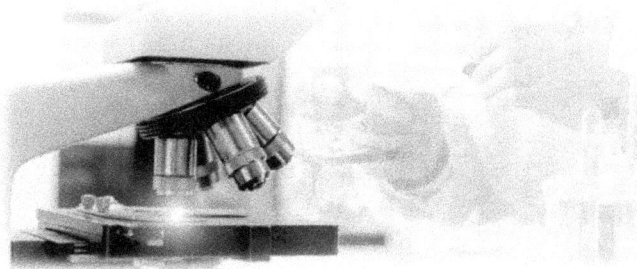

All vertebrate animals, including humans, are born with an Endocannabinoid System. The system consists of three components: endocannabinoids, the receptors which send and receive them, and the enzymes which break them down. Let's examine each of these three components.

Endocannabinoids

Endocannabinoids are chemical signals produced internally, which regulate function and keep our bodies running smoothly.

Anandamide is the most commonly known of the two endocannabinoids. Named for the Sanskrit term "Ananda," which means bliss, **anandamide produces a feeling of well-being.** Not surprisingly, anandamide is often called "The Bliss Molecule."

Until recently, we believed the phenomenon known as the "Runner's High" was caused by the release of adrenaline. However, after the discovery of the ECS, researchers now know that anandamide is responsible for this phenomenon.[29]

Unfortunately, the effects of anandamide are often short-lived as the compound is easily broken down and quickly metabolized by enzymes.

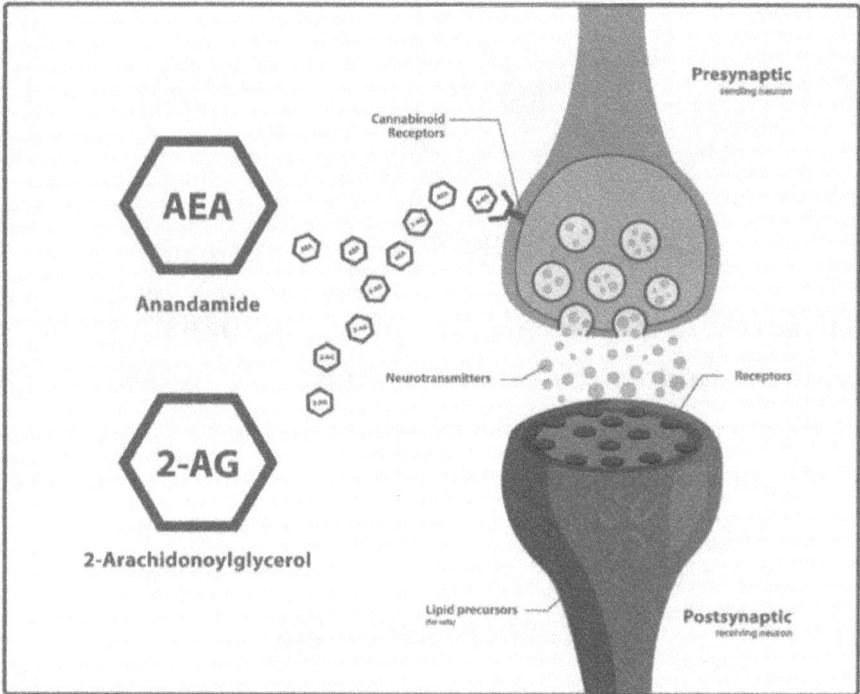

The second endocannabinoid is called 2-AG, or arachidonoyl-glycerol. **This chemical compound is considered a messenger molecule that plays a role in regulating signal transmission across synapses in the brain.**

Additional research suggests 2-AG is also responsible for the regulation of food intake and energy metabolism, as well as controlling mental disorders such as depression, anxiety, and addiction. 2-AG also helps maintain the inflammatory response and mitigation of pain.

Endocannabinoid Receptors

Endocannabinoid receptors are made of a protein chain that

wraps around cells inside the cell membrane. Acting like tiny antennas, receptors monitor the surrounding environment and send and receive chemical signals which tell cells how to respond.

Immune Cell   Neuron

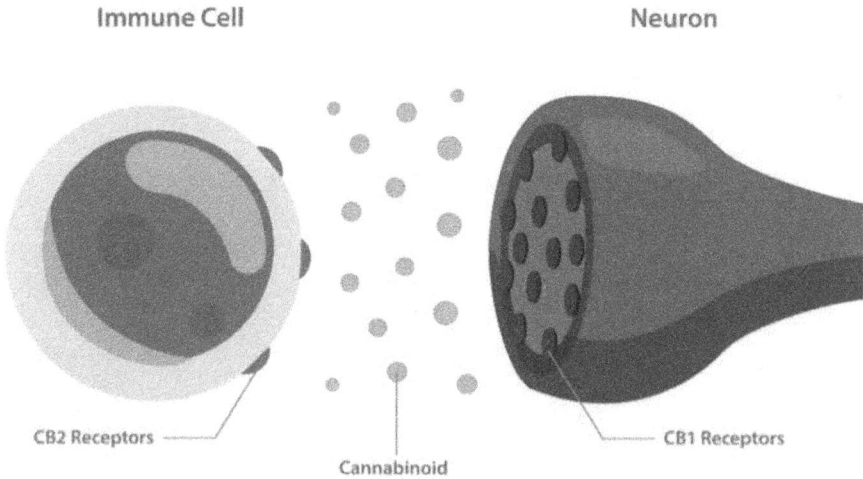

CB2 Receptors

Cannabinoid

CB1 Receptors

The two primary receptors in our body which receive endocannabinoids are called CB1 and CB2. Although similar in nature, these receptors have very different functions.

CB1

CB1 Receptors target:

- Motor activity
- Thinking
- Motor co-ordination
- Appetite
- Short term memory
- Pain perception
- Immune cells

CB2

CB2 Receptors are much broader than CB1 and influence most of the body

- Gut
- Kidneys
- Pancreas
- Adipose tissue
- Skeletal muscle
- Bone
- Eye
- Tumours
- Reproductive system
- Immune system
- Respiratory tract
- Skin
- CNS
- Cardiovascular system
- Liver

Metabolic Enzymes

The third and final component to the ECS is the metabolic enzymes that break down the chemical messengers after they've been used. Just as there are two endocannabinoids, there are two primary enzymes that metabolize them: FAAH and MAGL.

FAAH breaks down anandamide, while MAGL breaks down 2-AG. Unlike other hormones and neurotransmitters in the body, which can be stored and used later, enzymes in the endocannabinoid system degrade excessive cannabinoids that aren't needed. So, endocannabinoids are produced and metabolized on-demand.

Because these metabolic enzymes break down endogenous cannabinoids so efficiently, they often don't reach their full therapeutic potential. CBD has been shown to slow this process down by blocking the enzymes, allowing the natural cannabinoids to linger in the body longer.

Why the Endocannabinoid System Matters to You

The ultimate goal of the Endocannabinoid System is to keep the body in homeostasis. Homeostasis is defined as, "The process by which a living thing or a cell keeps the conditions inside it the same, despite any changes in the conditions around it." **In other words, the ECS helps our body find and maintain equilibrium and balance.**

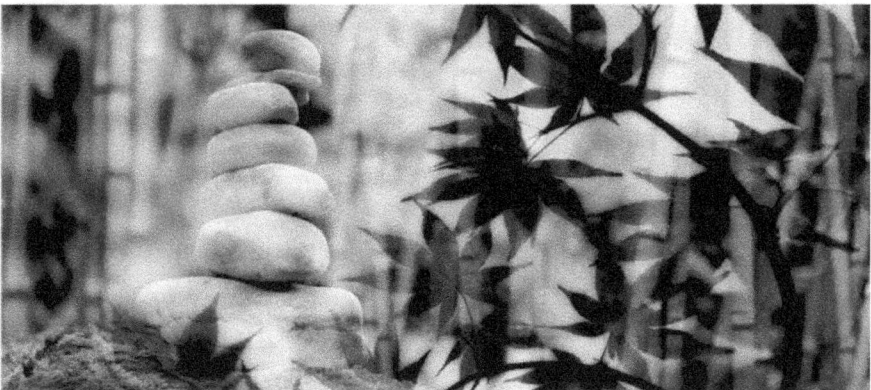

Research shows that to achieve perfect balance, the ECS inter-acts with all of the following physiological functions:[30]

- **Appetite & Digestion**
- **Metabolism**
- **Chronic Pain**
- **Inflammation**
- **Immune System Responses**
- **Mood & Stress**
- **Learning & Memory**
- **Motor Control**
- **Sleep**

- **Cardiovascular System Function**
- **Muscle Formation**
- **Bone Growth**
- **Liver Function**
- **Reproductive System Function**
- **Skin & Nerve Function**

Clearly, the ECS has a major impact on our overall health and well-being. But what happens when something goes awry, and the ECS can't reach homeostasis?

There is a condition known as Clinical Endocannabinoid Deficiency, or CED, which is defined by the body's inability to produce enough cannabinoids.

In 2003, Dr. Ethan Russo was the first to theorize that ECS deficiencies may be the root problem behind a multitude of ailments plaguing modern populations.[31]

Russo's findings show that migraines, fibromyal-

gia, and irritable bowel diagnosis are linked to Clinical Endocannabinoid Deficiency. There is also evidence that diabetic neuropathy, Huntington's disease, Multiple Sclerosis, and Parkinson's disease are also caused by CED as well.[32]

Dr. Russo believes that CBD supplementation may be the key to treating many of these chronic conditions, autoimmune disorders, and neurological diseases.

But Dr. Russo is not alone. In a study from the National Institute of Health, Pal Pacher and Geroge Kunos, leading scientists with the U.S. National Institutes of Health, made this statement,

> *"Modulating endocannabinoid system activity may have therapeutic potential in almost all diseases affecting humans, including obesity/metabolic syndrome, diabetes and diabetic complications, neurodegenerative, inflammatory, cardiovascular, liver, gastrointestinal, skin diseases, pain, psychiatric disorders, cachexia, cancer, chemotherapy-induced nausea and vomiting among many others."[33]*

CBD: Critical Support for the Most Important System in Your Body

As you can see, with ties to so many essential human functions, the ECS is one of the most critical systems in our bodies and quite possibly one of the most significant medical discoveries of the modern era. Logic tells us that ensuring our ECS operates at optimal levels is just as important as maintaining any of our other biological systems.

Today, it's universally understood that exercise supports the cardiovascular and respiratory systems; meditation nourishes the nervous system, and mindful nutrition protects the digestive system. So, it's easy to understand why millions of people from all over the world are now turning to CBD supplementation to maintain and nourish their Endocannabinoid System.

6

ALL-NATURAL CBD: A BETTER CHOICE THAN LAB-MADE PHARMACEUTICALS?

"I'm not here to wave the flag, but I do firmly believe that everyone should read up on the amazing CBD products that are coming out. Obviously, Big Pharma is probably not too pleased about all this arising from a simple plant God put in the ground."

— **Gene Simmons, Musician**

No one wants to start their day with a pharmaceutical cocktail. But according to statistics, the percentage of Americans (of all ages) taking five or more drugs nearly doubled from 8 percent to 15 percent between 2000 and 2012. **Shockingly, 46% of**

all people over the age of 70 take at least five pills per day.[34] While these statistics may seem high, doctors say it's not uncommon for older adults to take up to twenty prescriptions at once!

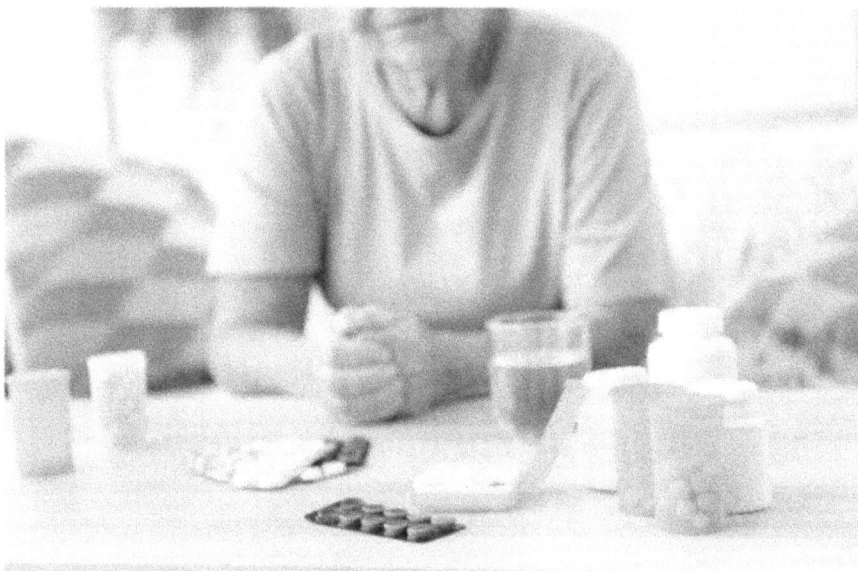

How did this happen? Over the last 50 years, the pharmaceutical industry shifted its primary focus from curing patient's ailments to maximizing company's profits.

Today, especially in the United States, it seems every time we turn on the television, there's another pharmaceutical commercial imploring us to "Ask your doctor!" Regardless of your symptoms, there's undoubtedly a pill for it:

- **Anxious? Take Prozac.**

- **Depressed? Take Effexor.**

- **Can't sleep? Take Ambien.**

- **Can't focus? Take Adderall.**

- **Have pain? Take Oxycontin.**

- **Nerve pain? Take Gabapentin.**

- **Muscle soreness? Take Flexeril.**

A Brief History of a Medical Travesty

"Everyday on TV there are commercials advertising the next best drug, and the second half of the commercial is all about the possible side effects. Well, I have never heard of a side effect from CBD."

– David Ahrens, NFL Athlete

The first television advertisement for a prescription medication was aired in 1983. A British pharmaceutical company named Boots created a television commercial for a pain reliever called Rufen.

This controversial first commercial created a wave of turmoil amongst regulators, policymakers, and the FDA. Even some pharmaceutical giants weighed in against direct-to-consumer advertisements. Edgar G. Davis, Vice President of Corporate Affairs for Eli Lilly and Company, stated,[35]

"We do not believe that commercial product advertising of prescription drugs is appropriate... prescription drugs embody a complex set of factors

with potential human effects that can best be evaluated by the physician... Therefore, we believe that the need for the physician's supervision of any prescription drug taken by the patient is paramount and that the potential pressures of public advertising of prescription drugs on the scientific decisions of the physician are both unwise and inappropriate."

However, under the guise of constitutional First Amendment rights to free speech, pharmaceutical companies prevailed in this debate and were granted permission to air their commercials. So the flood gates opened.

In 2017, the New York Times published an investigative story about the increase in pharmaceutical commercials on television. The newspaper cited data supplied by Kantar Media, revealing that over 770,000 advertisements were shown in 2016, an increase of almost 65 percent in just four years.[36] That's nearly 90 commercials an hour across all networks!

Did you know?

The United States and New Zealand are the only two countries in the world where pharmaceutical companies can advertise to the end-user?

Polypharmacy: The Devil Hidden in Plain Sight

Concurrent with the mass marketing of pharmaceuticals, we have witnessed the birth of a new trend called Polypharmacy.

Polypharmacy, in simple terms, is the use of more than one drug to treat a single medical condition. This happens when one drug causes unwanted side effects, so doctors prescribe another medication to control the adverse effects.

> *"It's very clear to me now that there is a much better and more sustainable way to manage what I call the recovery process... It doesn't matter who you are. We all have to manage these things to live a higher quality of life without taking a bunch of pharmaceuticals that typically create dependency and addiction."*
>
> – Riley Cote, NHL Athlete

But that's just the beginning! Polypharmacy compounds exponentially when medications prescribed for one ailment interact with medicines prescribed for another illness, creating an additional adverse condition, requiring yet another prescriptive cure. **Suddenly, the patient becomes trapped in an endless negative feedback loop of multiplying prescriptions that's impossible to escape.**

According to research published by Symbiosis, a journal of pharmacy and pharmaceutical sciences, as the number of conditions increases, the number of pills required to treat these ailments grows even faster.[37]

Statistics show that 15% of Seniors suffer a problem due to medication, of which more than half could've been prevented.[38]

Polypharmcy and Comorbidities

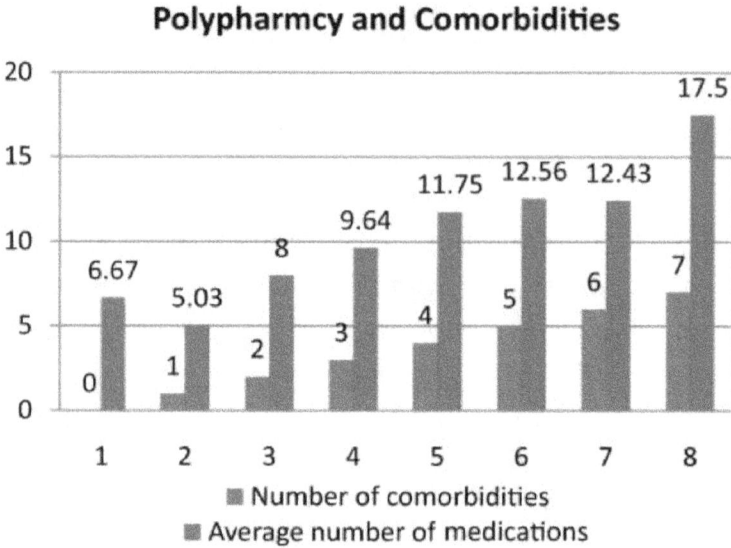

Bar chart showing Number of comorbidities and Average number of medications across categories 1 through 8:
- 1: 0 / 6.67
- 2: 1 / 5.03
- 3: 2 / 8
- 4: 3 / 9.64
- 5: 4 / 11.75
- 6: 5 / 12.56
- 7: 6 / 12.43
- 8: 7 / 17.5

■ Number of comorbidities
■ Average number of medications

Unintended Consequences of Polypharmacy

Multiple medications lead to numerous issues, including the following:

1. Lack of adherence.

Many older patients find it challenging to adhere to their prescribed regimen when given so many different drugs to maintain. This results in prescribed doses being inaccurately administered, or completely forgotten altogether. When this happens, medicines may not work the way they are expected. Physicians then prescribe additional drugs in a new attempt to achieve the original, desired results.

2. Too many doctors, too little communication.

Virtually all Seniors visit more than one doctor. Internists or specialists that treat specific conditions are often layered on top of general physicians. Many times, these doctors do not communicate with each other, leading to harmful interactions between medications.

3. The power of Big Pharma.

As unfortunate as it sounds, a significant reason why physicians prescribe so many drugs is purely for financial gain. Pharmaceutical companies have been under scrutiny for several years for their less than ethical sales practices that include kickbacks, lavish junkets and parties, and other schemes designed to encourage doctors to prescribe their products.

Everyone in today's modern society is familiar with the indecipherable, rapid-fire disclaimers that pharmaceutical companies squeeze into the last two seconds of their commercials. If you listen carefully, you will hear that Big Pharma admits that:

- Many medications for depression and mental illness can cause increased suicidal thoughts and tendencies – the very thing doctors prescribe them to prevent.

- Medications prescribed to induce sleep can cause sleepwalking so severe that the consumer may actually drive their car while still sleeping.

- Certain medications for mental illness might have caused men to grow breasts.

- Many, if not most, of the FDA-approved, heavily prescribed medications on the market today can cause death.

If these medications come with a mile-long list of side effects by themselves, imagine what combining them together does! Some may cancel each other out, ultimately providing no benefits to the consumer at all, while others may not interact well together and only make matters worse.

Imagine complimenting your entire medicine cabinet with a single, all natural, and affordable solution that's available in a variety of formulations to meet your specific tastes and needs. Sound miraculous? It is. **The solution is CBD.**

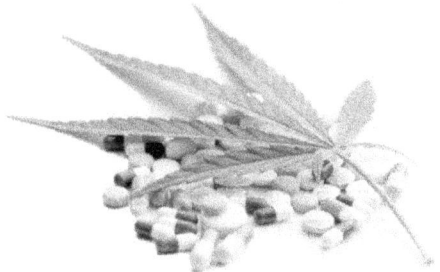

PART 2

SECRET CBD CURES
EVERY SENIOR SHOULD KNOW

Earlier in this book, I said CBD provides hope for those suffering from a whole host of ailments and conditions. A calm, restful life, free from stress and anxiety, may now be yours through CBD supplementation! **From chronic pain conditions to autoimmune disorders, neurological illnesses to mental health issues, people are finding relief through hemp derived, full spectrum, and broad spectrum CBD and its associated cannabinoids, terpenes, and flavonoids.**

Let's review the existing research and the actual success stories from patients that have found success with CBD supplementation.

This vital information will help you make an educated decision on how CBD can best benefit you and improve your life.

7

ANXIETY & MENTAL HEALTH

"CBD was to help soothe my anxiety. It was a huge relief for me to feel like myself, yet the edge was gone. The bonus of the whole thing was the relief from aches and pains. It immediately alleviated 90% of my pain."

— Tom Hanks, Actor

- Anxiety
- Depression
- Schizophrenia

- PTSD
- Mood Disorders
- Stress

Mental illness is a significant problem in the United States across all age groups. According to the National Institute of Mental Health, in 2017, more than 46 million people, or 18.9% of all adults have a mental health disorder.[39]

Despite 1 in 5 adults dealing with mental illness on some level, sadly, only 41 percent will receive mental health care services.[40] That's because stigma, shame, and embarrassment often prevent sufferers from seeking help. Long-term mental illness is tied to several severe, although treatable, medical conditions. Additionally, psychiatric diseases, such as depression and anxiety, often co-occur with the diagnosis of other chronic diseases.

In fact, according to CDC statistics,

- **23% of cardiovascular cases also deal with depression.**

- **27% of diabetic patients are diagnosed with depression.**

- **40% of cancer patients also develop depression.**

Not surprisingly, homicides, suicides, and even unintentional accidents are two to six times higher for people with mental illness.[41] Tragically, research suggests that adults with serious mental illness die 25 years earlier than other patients.[42]

Traditional treatments for mental illness include rigorous cognitive treatment and appointments with psychologists and psychiatrists. Many times, in addition to cognitive and behavioral therapies, a myriad of drug treatments are prescribed, including:

- Antidepressants – Effexor, Cymbalta, Lexapro
- Anti-anxiolytics – Xanax, Ativan
- Mood Stabilizers – Lithium, Tegretol
- Anti-psychotics – Seroquel, Abilify, Latuda

Polypharmacy Rears Its Ugly Head

Counterintuitively, the medications listed above often come with a broad range of adverse side effects including:

- Low Blood Sugar
- Low Sodium
- Nausea/ Stomach Issues
- Constipation/ Diarrhea
- Insomnia
- Headaches
- Tremors
- Sexual Dysfunction
- Increased Anxiety
- Suicide Ideation
- Apathy
- Irregular Heartbeat
- High Blood Pressure
- Blurred Vision
- Seizures
- Weight Loss/ Gain

As we've previously discussed, these side effects lead to additional prescriptions, which results in compounding the patient's original medical problems.

CBD: Your All-Natural Solution for Mental Health Disorders

Mental illnesses often start as a result of inflammation and the malfunctioning of chemical signals in the brain, such as serotonin, dopamine, and glutamate. These chemical signals are responsible for our overall feelings of well-being and happiness.

Let's review how these different signals work and how CBD may positively affect them:

Serotonin

Serotonin helps control our mood, sex drive, appetite, and sleep. Low serotonin contributes to anxiety and depressive symptoms. Often physicians prescribe SSRIs (selective serotonin reuptake inhibitors) to increase the level of serotonin in the brain. Unfortunately, these drugs tell the receptors there's enough serotonin, so the body stops producing serotonin on its own.

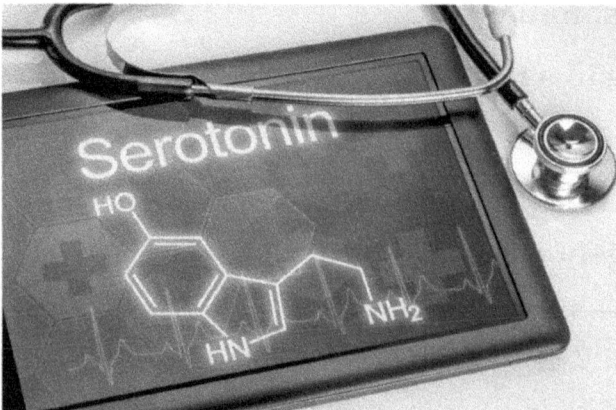

CBD works differently than SSRIs. CBD boosts the functionality of serotonin receptors without inhibiting the production of serotonin.[43] Gabriella Gobbi, a neuroscientist and psychiatrist, explains how CBD moderates the serotonin response: "After a few days, you get this sensitization of 5-HT1A, as you would with an SSRI, and increased serotonin signaling."[44]

Dopamine

In anxiety disorders, the brain does not have the right level of dopamine. Studies indicate that too much dopamine could contribute to increased anxiety.[45] **CBD has the potential to modulate how dopamine is released,** thus having promise as an anti-psychotic.

GABA

GABA works as a calming agent, controlling over-stimulated neurons and relaxing muscles. Low GABA increases anxiety symptoms and nervousness. **CBD inhibits the reabsorption of GABA, so it can build up and quiet over-stimulated neurons.**

Glutamate

Glutamate is an essential neurotransmitter in the brain, which plays a part in memory and learning, as well as our stress and fear response. Glutamate influences how we develop and maintain fear and is connected to both anxiety and depression symptoms.[46,47] By binding with adenosine receptors, **CBD can regulate how neurons release glutamate and dopamine.**[48]

Additionally, there are other ways CBD and other cannabinoids may assist with mental health conditions. Interacting with a broad range of receptors in the brain and body, CBD has multiple pathways to help calm over-excited neurons and help minimize mental illness symptoms.

- **CBD reduces hypothalamic activity.** Stress causes increased activity in the hypothalamus. Reducing this activity can reduce anxiety symptoms.[49]

- **CBD inhibits the uptake of norepinephrine**, which heightens arousal, alertness, and boosts concentration and attention.[50]

- **CBD inhibits FAAH enzymes,** which breakdown anandamide, thus increasing the levels of the endocannabinoid.[51]

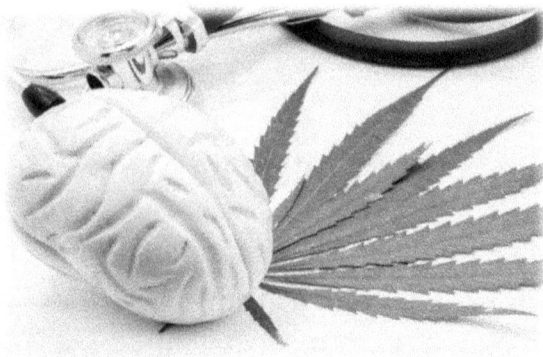

CBD & Mental Health: The Research is Compelling

While more research is undoubtedly welcomed, several small clinical trials and animal models have provided the following positive results:

- In a 2011 clinical trial studying social anxiety, some patients with anxiety were given CBD, while others were given a placebo, and all were asked to perform a task. Those who received a placebo for their anxiety experienced no change. However, those who received CBD performed similarly to the healthy control group without anxiety.[52]

- Other studies show similar results. Two double-blind studies from 2010 concluded CBD significantly reduced anxiety symptoms in human patients.[53]

What Patients are Saying

Every day, people from all walks of life report that using CBD oil helps tremendously with anxiety. I can personally attest to these amazing claims.

Previous to my personal CBD supplementation, I was on a rollercoaster ride of experimentation that led me to experiment with over a dozen prescription SSRIs. **Once CBD sup-**

plementation was introduced into my life, the debilitating cloud of anxiety and worry that always hovered over me quickly lifted.

Additionally, my collaborator Kristina Etter, will tell you that during 20 years in a high-stress career, anxiety and depression were an ever-present part of her daily life. Each day, Kristina relied heavily on multiple SSRI medications and benzodiazepines for anxiety. These drugs caused a mental fog, fatigue, and drowsiness, which only exacerbated matters and negatively affected her performance.

Yet again, polypharmacy reared its ugly head, as doctors prescribed Ritalin and Adderall, powerful amphetamines, to counter the nasty side effects of Kristina's original prescriptions. This led to a negative feedback loop as the new drugs ultimately diminished any therapeutic impact from the originally prescribed medications.

While it took a little time to find the right combination of cannabinoids, Kristina soon found consistent symptom relief with none of the side effects of the dangerous and expensive pharmaceutical cocktail she used previously.

Like the two of us, **millions of other people have found CBD supplementation to help with anxiety, depression, and a whole list of other mental illnesses.** Here are just a few testimonials of benefits that may be available to you:

ANXIETY

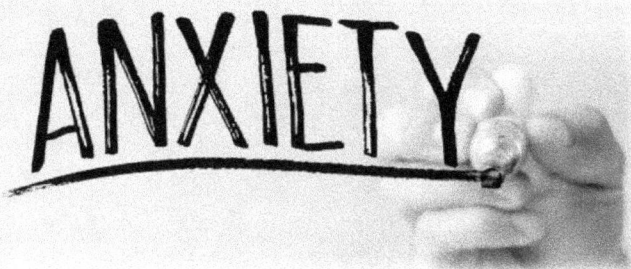

In 2019, Quartz ran a survey of more than 2,000 Americans. Of those who answered, 55 percent claimed to use CBD for relaxation, and 50 percent said they use CBD specifically for stress and anxiety.[54]

"The biggest killer on the planet is stress and I still think the best medicine is and always has been cannabis."

– Willie Nelson, Musician

"After about a month of ingesting a 10-milligram dose of CBD tincture under my tongue twice a day, I gradually felt a sense of calm and relaxation. From there, I slowly weaned down off of my anxiety prescription."

– Newsweek

"CBD's subtle calming nature helped with my anxiety."[55]

– Riley Cote, NHL Athlete

"I have observed first-hand the life changing benefits of CBD for my Senior clients struggling with depression, anxiety, and chronic pain."

– Tammy Fried, LCSW

8

CHRONIC PAIN CONDITIONS

"A bonus of CBD was the relief from various aches and pains. Especially the arthritis in my knees. It immediately alleviated 90% of my pain. The benefits of CBD are unlike anything any pill or medication can do."

— Tom Hanks, Actor

- **Inflammatory Pain**

- **Arthritis**

- **Osteoarthritis**

- **Spinal Stenosis**

- **Degenerative Disc Disease**

- **Gout**

- **Plantar Fasciitis**

- **Migraines**

Chronic pain conditions plague the United States. A study published by the CDC concluded,[56] "In 2016, an estimated 20.4% of U.S. adults had chronic pain, and 8.0% of U.S. adults had high-impact chronic pain, with higher prevalence associated with advancing age."

Traditional treatments for chronic pain almost always include opioid-based medications. A report published by the CDC in 2017 indicates that the number of opioids prescribed per person is around three times higher than it was in 1999.[57] In fact, the report shows that physicians write more than 58 opioid prescriptions for every 100 Americans.

Unfortunately, another report from 2017 suggests that people over the age of 65 make up more than 25 percent of long-term opiate consumers.[58] While opiates may be appropriate in triage and short-term situations, long-term opioid use can be hazardous and detrimental.

Opioid Use Often Results in Addiction and Death

According to the American Addiction Centers website,[59] a regular regimen of opioids in the long-term can cause severe problems, including:

- **Nausea & Vomiting**
- **Stomach Distention & Bloating**
- **Constipation**
- **Dependence**

- **Development of Tolerance** (requiring more and more to get the same level of pain relief)

- **Liver Damage** (especially with drugs combining opiates with acetaminophen)

- **Brain Damage** (due to oxygen deficiency due to respiratory depression)

And even... **Death.**

(Due to accidental overdose, respiratory failure, or organ failure)

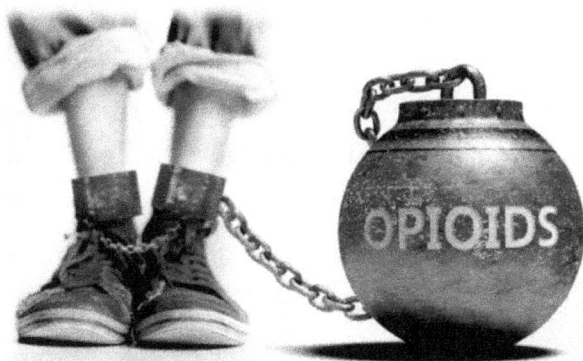

In addition to opioid medications, doctors also frequently prescribe NSAIDs or non-steroidal anti-inflammatory drugs such as aspirin and ibuprofen. Long-term use of these kinds of drugs can lead to stomach ulcers, kidney and liver failure, and GI bleeding, all of which are potentially fatal. In fact, current research estimates that the number of deaths per year due to NSAIDs ranges from 3,500[60] to more than 16,000[61] depending on the study.

Because of all these problems, it should be no surprise that **pain is the number one reason people use CBD today.** A report published in early 2019 surveyed registered cannabis patients across the United States and found that nearly 65 percent of patients consume cannabis for chronic pain conditions.[62]

CBD: Your All-Natural Solution for Pain

Let's look at how CBD battles pain, and why so many people call it a miracle medicine.

In chapter five, we talked about the endocannabinoid system and its ability to regulate and control various systems within our bodies. One of those functions was pain perception.

For example, when you stub your toe, your body releases pain-causing chemicals, proinflammatory cells, and neurotransmitters, which ultimately trigger the release of endocannabinoids to control the pain response.[63] By learning how to manipulate certain functions of the ECS, researchers believe we may be able to alter how our body responds to pain.

How CBD Works to Reduce Your Pain

- **Reduces Inflammation** – Inflammation control is one of the best-known benefits of CBD. Cannabinoids work to suppress the natural inflammation response by controlling and suppressing specific inflammatory cells and even causing a controlled cell death, known as apoptosis, to active inflammatory cells.[64]

- **CB2 Receptor Activation** – By activating these receptors, CBD helps the ECS control the inflammatory response by decreasing cytokines or the body's pro-inflammatory cells. More cytokines increase pain and contribute to chronic pain conditions.[65]

- **Activates Non-Cannabinoid Receptors** – Besides the ECS receptors, CBD activates other receptors, such as adenosine,[66] vanilloid,[67] serotoin,[68] and PPAR receptors[69] – all of which are associated with pain and inflammation.

- **Stimulates Opioid Receptors** – CBD can positively alter opioid receptors and how they function to reduce pain production.[70]

- **Increases Anandamide** – CBD improves the body's natural anandamide levels by binding with specific enzymes and proteins, which ultimately extends the life of anandamide, so it has more time to work its magic on the endocannabinoid system.[71]

CBD & Pain: The Research is Compelling

Much of the research into cannabis and CBD thus far has been done on lab animals. While animal studies may not translate to human results, they certainly provide a starting point for clinical research. Additionally, we can look at clinical trials for synthetic cannabinoids such as Sativex.

Sativex is a synthetic cannabinoid pharmaceutical product which contains 2.7mg of THC and 2.5mg of CBD, or a 1:1 ratio of cannabinoids. Synthetic simply means it was made in a laboratory setting rather than extracted from the plant.

Although not approved in the United States, Sativex has been approved in 25 other countries. Canada approved Sativex for neuropathic pain in 2005 and for cancer pain in 2007. Additionally, there have been numerous clinical trials using Sativex for neuropathic pain, rheumatoid arthritis, and cancer pain. Here are just a few studies to date:

- **Neuropathic Pain** – Half of 125 trial participants, used a 1:1 THC to CBD formula and reported significant improvement in pain levels compared to other participants who received a placebo.[72]

- **Intractable Cancer Pain** – 177 cancer patients either received a dose of CBD/THC, just THC, or a placebo. The group receiving the CBD/THC blend reported a significant improvement in pain.[73]

- **Rheumatoid Arthritis** – 31 participants with RA were given Sativex, while 27 were given a placebo. Those using Sativex reported a substantial reduction in pain intensity and improved quality of life.[74]

- **Spinal Cord Injury** – Vaping cannabis proved to reduce pain symptoms compared to placebo in a study of 42 patients with spinal cord injuries and diseases.[75]

- **HIV/AIDS** – A survey of 178 HIV patients showed that inhaled cannabis improves peripheral neuropathy.[76]

- **Migraine** – Between 2010 and 2014, researchers tracked 121 consumers using cannabis for migraine headaches. Headache frequency reduced from more than 10 per month to less than 5.[77]

- **Fibromyalgia** – In 2011, a study of 56 patients with fibromyalgia showed cannabis improved pain intensity, reduced stiffness, a sense of relaxation, and an improvement in overall well-being.[78]

What Patients are Saying

"I enjoyed a 10-year playing career. I have taken more pain pills in that time than most people have in their lifetime… in the beginning of my career, it was handed out like candy. I wish I had known about the benefits of CBD much earlier."

– David Ahrens, NFL Athlete

"Recently I did a play on Broadway for six months. My body was wrecked, [and] my neck was really tight. The CBD has relaxing benefits, and the idea is to avoid using too many painkillers."

– Olivia Wilde, Actor

"I've been on CBD for well over a year now, and I can tell you that my body feels great. I have no more inflammation in my body, my knee, and my joint pain is gone. My migraines – I haven't taken migraine medicine for over a year."

– Terrell Davis, NFL Athlete

"I started taking CBD oil and that is when it really happened, like wow, the pain went away. I can get

down and play with Legos on the floor with my kids. And if my wife says, 'hey can you get me some water? I'm like boom! I just up, run over, get water and run back."

— Jake Plummer, NFL Athlete

9

SLEEP

"A small but growing body of scientific research provides some support for CBD as a sleep aid. About 10% of Americans who reported trying CBD said they used it to help them sleep, and a majority of those people said it worked."

— Consumer Reports

Sleep is absolutely critical for good health and a high quality of life.

However, according to a nationally representative Consumer Reports survey, almost 80% of all Americans say they have trouble sleeping at least once a week.[79] **Sleeping can be even more challenging for older adults, with more than half suffering regularly from insomnia.**

This lack of sleep comes with severe costs and repercussions. Without regular rest, the body simply stops functioning properly, ultimately causing a wide range of health risks.

Complications of Insomnia

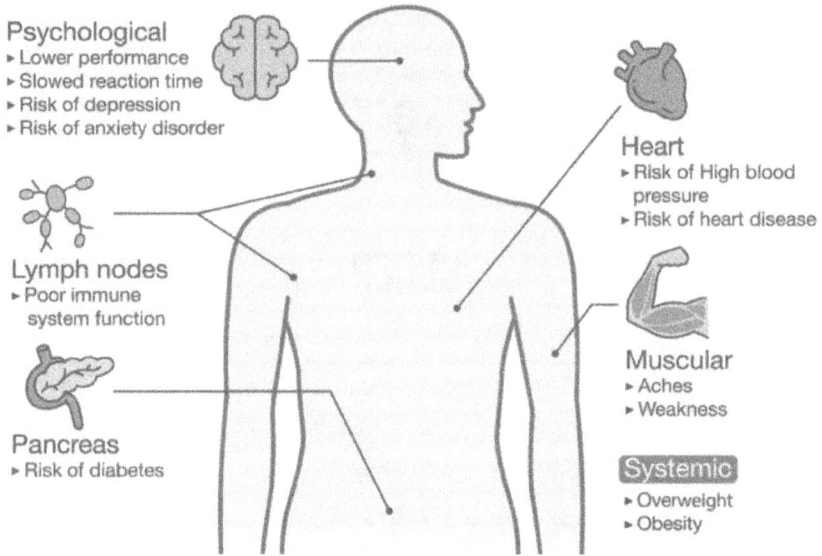

Psychological
▸ Lower performance
▸ Slowed reaction time
▸ Risk of depression
▸ Risk of anxiety disorder

Lymph nodes
▸ Poor immune
  system function

Pancreas
▸ Risk of diabetes

Heart
▸ Risk of High blood
  pressure
▸ Risk of heart disease

Muscular
▸ Aches
▸ Weakness

Systemic
▸ Overweight
▸ Obesity

Unfortunately, for some people, no matter how hard they try to naturally improve their sleep (through hacks like increased exercise and decreased screen time), sleep still escapes them, eventually necessitating a visit to their physician, and of course, yet another prescription medication.

The side effects caused by most prescription drugs for insomnia are amongst the most debilitating on the market. While Rosanne Barr may have caused everyone to scratch their heads when she claimed Ambien caused her deplorable behavior online, unbelievably, she might not be too far from the truth.

In March of 2009, a 45-year-old man walked into his estranged wife's place of work and opened fire. He killed eight people and wounded two others. Yet, the defense team successfully argued that the man was under the influence of Ambien at the time, thus getting his conviction reduced from first-degree murder to second-degree murder.[80]

The Truth About Sleep Aids and Their Side Effects

While committing felony murder isn't a common side effect of these drugs, there are many disturbing side effects that accompany prescription sleep medications, including:

- Burning or tingling in the extremities
- Appetite changes
- Constipation
- Diarrhea
- Balance issues
- Dizziness
- Daytime drowsiness

- Dry mouth or throat
- Flatulence
- Headaches
- Heartburn/Indigestion
- Impairment
- Mental slowing or problems with attention or memory

- **Stomach pain or tenderness**
- **Uncontrollable shaking of a part of the body**

- **Unusual dreams**
- **Weakness**

Unfortunately, this isn't an exhaustive list of side effects. Sleep medicines can also cause parasomnias or movements, behaviors, and actions that occur while you're still asleep. During these episodes, you have no self-control, like sleepwalking, sleep-eating, or even sleep-driving!

CBD: Your All Natural Solution for Sleep

As mentioned earlier in Chapter 5, the Endocannabinoid System is a relatively new medical discovery, and although research is picking up pace, there's still much to learn. While we know the ECS is most definitely involved in modulating our sleep/wake cycles, or circadian rhythm, the actual mechanism of its involvement is still up for debate.

To explain, let's first define a couple of pharmacology terms.

- **Agonist** - An agonist is defined as a chemical, hormone, drug, or substance which binds to a receptor activating it to elicit a biological response.

- **Antagonist** – On the other hand, an antagonist blocks the action of the agonist.

In this case, researchers agree that CB1 is the endocannabinoid receptor found in our brain and central nervous system. We also know that anandamide is a natural agonist of the CB1 receptor, whereas 2-AG is an antagonist.[81]

Similarly, we know that THC acts as an agonist with the CB1 receptor, while CBD is an antagonist of the same receptor. In other words, **THC activates the CB1 receptor, while CBD prevents the receptor from being activated.**

However, here's where the science starts to fracture as compared to what consumers are reporting. According to research, activating the CB1 receptor induces sleep. Therefore, a CB1 antagonist (in this case, CBD) should induce wakefulness. Yet, thousands of people report that CBD is helping them get a better night's sleep. So, how can this be? Allow me to share two possible explanations:

Explanation #1 – The Source of Insomnia

Many people are sleep deprived because of other chronic conditions, such as pain or anxiety. For many people, shutting off the spinning gears in their mind or quelling their pain is next to impossible and they end up staring at the ceiling all night.

Since CBD works so well at silencing the anxious voices and reducing pain and inflammation, I suspect that many people who report miraculous sleep benefits from CBD are actually treating the underlying anxiety that is keeping them awake at night.

Explanation #2 – The Entourage Effect

We know that other cannabinoids, terpenes, and flavonoids from the plant can alter the effects. So, in full and broad spectrum CBD oils, you're not getting just CBD – you're getting small amounts of other compounds such as CBN, myrcene, or linalool. All of these compounds have been found in studies to be relaxing and sedative.

This theory is supported by research. An Israeli cannabis producer and research facility, Kanabo Research, recently published results from a pre-clinical trial they conducted on various formulations of cannabinoids for sleep as compared to diazepam (Valium). **Their research concluded that a combination of CBD, CBN, and either myrcene or linalool produced longer-lasting sleep than the pharmaceuticals.**[82]

CBD & Sleep: The Research is Compelling

As of now, researchers are still examining CBD's role in sleep regulation, but here are a few studies revealing its potential abilities to assist with sleep:

- Chronic Pain/Sleep – Researchers studied 2000 subjects with chronic pain and sleep disorders. The Sativex 1:1 ratio product significantly improved both pain perception and sleep issues.[83]

- In a 2013 study, researchers assessed CBD's ability of treating sleep disorders in rats. They found that the rats treated with CBD slept more than the rats who received a placebo, suggesting CBD can increase total sleep time and sleep latency.[84]

- A 2019 study on CBD for sleep and anxiety found that 66.7% of the 72 individuals treated with CBD slept better for the first month, though effectiveness diminished over time.[85]

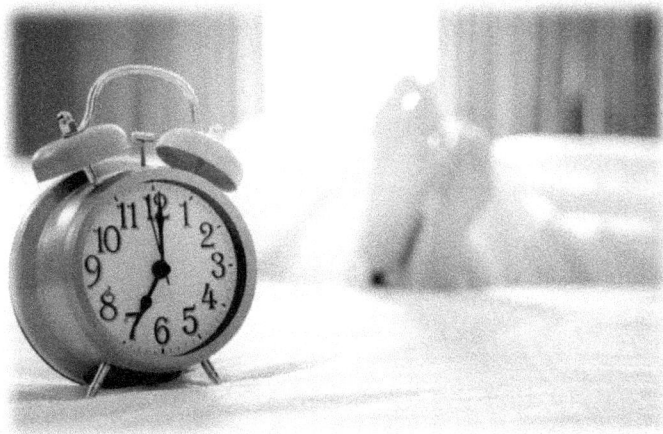

What Patients are Saying

"It just calms you... CBD oil is much better than sleeping pills."

— Roger Daltrey, Musician

"I'm getting older and I have inflammation in my body. I'm waking up with better sleep."

— Bubba Watson, PGA Athlete

"I quickly realized it wasn't just helping with my brain health, but it also added another dimension to my sleep."

— Riley Cote, NHL Athlete

"I have been taking CBD oil for the last 2 years for chronic neck pain as well as for a sleep aid."

— Lauren Lockey, Health & Wellness Expert

10

CANCER

"I kicked cancer's ass with CBD."

— Tommy Chong, Comedian

- **Lung Cancer**
- **Leukemia**
- **Breast Cancer**
- **Brain Cancer**
- **Pancreatic Cancer**
- **Colon Cancer**

Everyone's life has been affected by cancer in one way or another. More than 1.7 million new cases of cancer were diagnosed in 2018, and more than 600,000 people die from cancer each year. In fact, according to the National Cancer Institute, more than 1 in 3 people in the United States will get some form of cancer during their lives.[86]

Age is the Single Biggest Risk Factor for Cancer

The facts show the risk of being diagnosed with cancer increases significantly after age 50. **Half of all cancers occur at age 66 and above,** and according to the National Cancer Institute, one-quarter of all new cancer diagnoses occur in people between the ages of 65 and 74.

Traditional treatments for cancer are highly destructive. If feasible, a surgeon will likely perform surgery to remove as much of the tumor as possible. After surgery, a regimen of chemotherapy and radiation therapies is often prescribed to kill any remaining cancer cells. These treatments frequently come with extreme side effects as these are lethal solutions that often kill healthy cells along with the cancer cells.

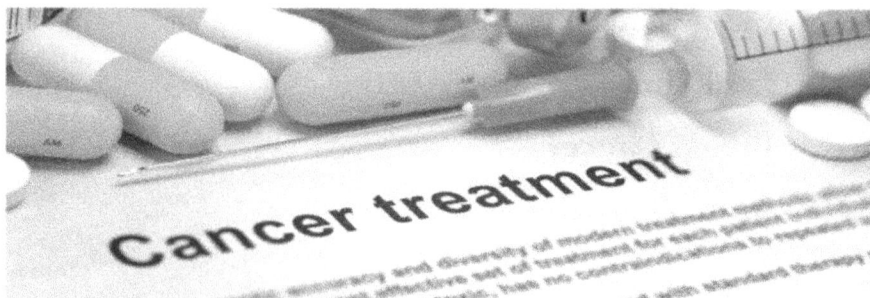

Side effects for chemotherapy and radiation include:[87]

- Anemia
- Appetite Loss
- Bleeding and Bruising
- Constipation
- Delirium
- Diarrhea
- Edema (Swelling)
- Fatigue
- Fertility Issues
- Flu-Like Symptoms
- Hair Loss
- Infection and Neutropenia
- Lymphedema
- Memory and Concentration Problems
- Mouth & Throat Problems
- Nausea and Vomiting
- Nerve Problems
- Organ-Related Inflammation and Immunotherapy
- Pain
- Sexual Health Issues
- Skin/Nail Changes
- Sleep Problems
- Urinary/Bladder Problems

Long-term side effects of cancer treatments can include problems with kidney function, fertility issues, impotence, secondary tumors, gastrointestinal issues, as well as issues with the thyroid, liver (hepatitis), and heart (heart attacks).

To treat the side effects of these invasive treatments, physicians prescribe additional medications, presenting an opportunity for polypharmacy and overmedication yet again.

How the ECS is Involved

Cancer is caused when abnormal cells essentially hide from your immune system. As these cells continue to divide and multiply, they build up and a mass or tumor forms. Since the Endocannabinoid System is intertwined with our immune system, some researchers and physicians believe that learning how to modulate the ECS may help in the prevention and treatment of certain types of cancer.[88]

Activating the ECS may slow the proliferation of cancer cells and help keep them from migrating to other parts of the body, as well as, induce apoptosis, or controlled cell death.

CBD: An All-Natural Way to Battle Cancer?

Unfortunately, naturally produced endocannabinoids are easily degraded within the body, so their effects are short-lived. This is why phytocannabinoids may prove to be beneficial, as more research begins to unfold. Here are a few ways researchers believe CBD may hold a valuable key to cancer treatment:

Apoptosis

Cells die in our bodies all the time. However, destructive cell death, or necrosis, is when trauma causes certain cells to explode, leaving harmful proteins and debris floating around in the tissues. Apoptosis is different. The cell dies, but it doesn't explode and leave a mess. A cleanup cell, called a macrophage, comes by later and removes the dead cell.

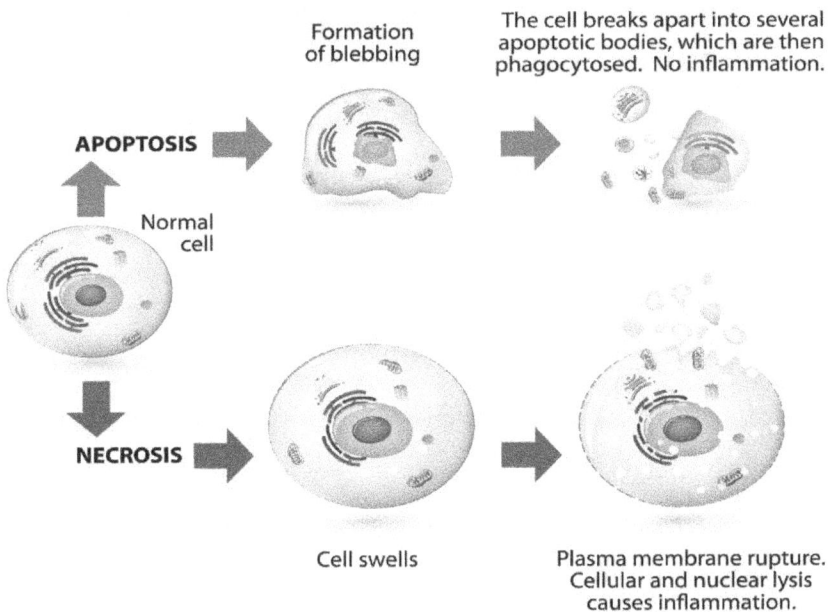

Apoptosis Compared to Necrosis

Chemo and radiation kill everything in its path, including healthy cells, which is why so many patients get sick during these treatments. By activating specific pathways,[89] CBD can lead cancer cells into a natural death process. **Unlike chemo and radiation, activation of these pathways with CBD** only causes trauma to the cancer cells and leaves the healthy cells alone.

Angiogenesis

A natural process in the body to form new blood vessels, angiogenesis is an essential process for healthy growth and development. Unfortunately, angiogenesis also contributes to cancer growth and proliferation. As the blood vessels form, they provide the nutrients that cancer needs to run rampant, growing and multiplying until it invades other parts of the body.

Once cancer cells reach the vascular and lymphatic systems, they can travel to new locations anywhere in the body. Once they invade other parts of the body, angiogenesis starts again, and the cancer cells grow in new areas.

Research has shown CBD can inhibit angiogenesis in a couple of ways.[90] **By binding with specific receptors, CBD reduces oxidative stress[91] and affects pathways known for regulating how cancer develops.[92]**

Besides inducing apoptosis and slowing angiogenesis, research also suggests **CBD may control the expression of particular genes that control the spread of cancer.** Studies have revealed a specific gene that is present in more than 20 different types of cancer.[93]

Anandamide

This is a natural cannabinoid produced within the body that has been shown to have potent anti-cancer effects. Research suggests that anandamide slows cancer cell growth[94] and induces apoptosis in cancer cells, which have become resistant.[95]

Additionally, particularly in breast cancer, researchers have found that high prolactin may increase the risk. Anandamide can suppress prolactin.[96]

As we've discussed in previous conditions, CBD can increase the amount of anandamide in the body by binding with the proteins and enzymes that breakdown and consume anandamide.[97]

CBD & Cancer: The Research is Compelling

Research regarding the effects of cannabinoids on cancer has been ongoing for decades. **From all corners of the globe, researchers are finding that cannabinoids may hold the keys to unlocking a cure for cancer.** Let's review a few studies involving CBD and cancer.

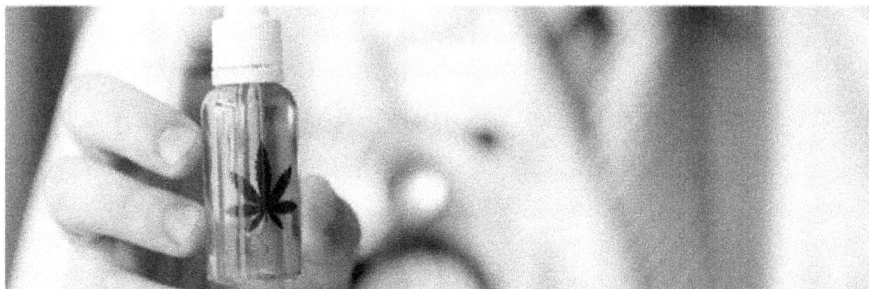

Brain Cancer

In a 2004 laboratory study, CBD was added to human glioma cells, resulting in reduced proliferation and apoptosis. Researchers have also observed similar results in mice.[98]

Breast Cancer

Research was published in 2007, testing different cannabinoids and other synthetics on human breast cancer cells. The results showed CBD as the most potent cannabinoid against cancer cell proliferation, migration, and invasion.[99]

Cervical Cancer

A report published in 2016 looked for evidence that cannabis sativa extract could help treat cervical cancer. The tests not only showed that cannabis has positive results against cancer, but that CBD, in particular, induced apoptosis of cancer cells.[100]

Colorectal Cancer

Research in 2016 revealed that by activating CB1 and CB2 endocannabinoid receptors, CBD was able to decrease colorectal cancer proliferation. Researchers also noted that despite the efficiency of inhibiting cancer growth, CBD did not impact any of the healthy cells and tissues surrounding the area.[101]

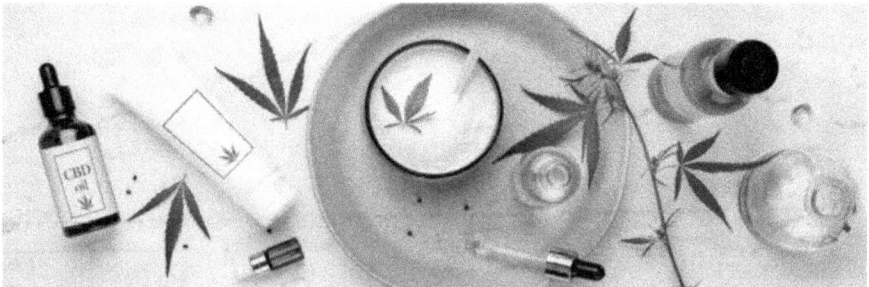

Leukemia

Much research has been done on cannabinoids and leukemia. A study was published by researchers in 1975, showing THC and CBD both having an impact on cancerous cells in leukemia and lung cancer.[102]

Another study out of the University of London, Oxford published more than 40 years later in the International Journal of Oncology, showed similar results.[103]

Lung Cancer

A study from 2010 indicates CBD slows the invasion of certain types of lung cancer cells. Further research from 2010 also suggests CB1 and CB2 receptors as possible targets for slowing the growth of non-small cell lung cancer, as well.[104]

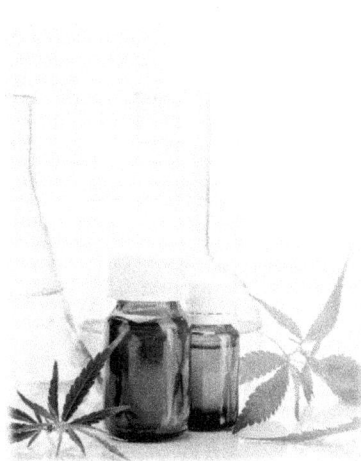

Prostate Cancer

A study published in 2014 showed CBD could down-regulate, or decrease, the number of receptors, as well as decrease the production of prostate antigens.[105]

What Patients are Saying

Many people today can tell stories of cancer survival, and many of them are telling a story of cannabis alongside more traditional treatments. Celebrities from the United States and around the globe are among those who've begun to sing the praises of cannabis for cancer.

Although still battling the disease, Olivia Newton-John, is open about her cannabis use. The 70-year-old actress and singer recently appeared on an episode of 60-Minutes to discuss her treatment approach using a host of alternative treatments such as cannabis oil, acupuncture, meditation, and other herbal remedies prepared by her husband.

11

NEUROLOGICAL DISEASES

"CBD acts as an antioxidant and neuroprotector for the brain in relation to concussions."

— Marvin Washington, NFL Athlete

- Huntington's Disease
- Parkinson's Disease
- Multiple Sclerosis
- Alzheimer's Disease
- Stroke
- ALS
- Epilepsy
- Dementia

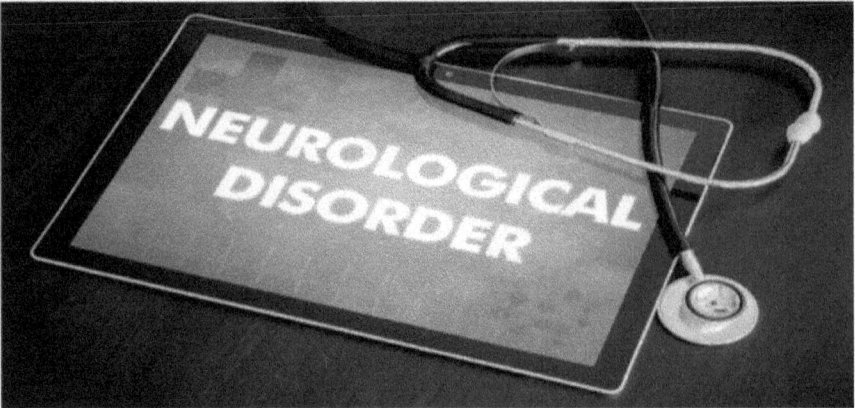

The American Neurological Association reports that around 100 million Americans are diagnosed with at least one of more than 1,000 neurological conditions.[106] Neurological disorders negatively affect the brain, spine, and central nervous system.

Issues in the nervous system can cause difficulties with basic human tasks such as learning, moving, speaking, swallowing, and even breathing! The range of symptoms that neurological conditions cause includes:

- **Tremors**

- **Chronic Pain**

- **Muscle Weakness**

- **Seizures**

- **Paralysis**
  (*Partial or Complete*)

- **Loss of Sensation**

- **Troubles Reading & Writing**

- **Cognitive Decline**

- **Unexplained Pain**

- **Decreased Alertness**

Because this range of symptoms is so diverse, the opportunity for polypharmacy pops up yet again. Physicians prescribe a variety of pharmaceuticals to control these symptoms. Additionally, physical therapy and/or physiotherapy is often prescribed to help maintain or restore function. Cognitive therapy may also help with anxiety and other mood disorders associated with neurological disorders. But, as with the other conditions we have already discussed, these mental side effects are often treated with yet another prescription.

How the ECS is Involved

Most neurological conditions are degenerative diseases and result from the death of neurons in the brain. Inflammation also plays a vital role in the development of many neurological disorders. Additionally, malfunctions in neurotransmitters (dopamine, serotonin, and glutamate) contribute to the development of specific neurodegenerative conditions as well.

Because the ECS is continuously looking for balance, manipulating how the receptors respond may prove beneficial in most, if not all, neurological conditions.

In Parkinson's disease, there is a slow but progressive reduction in dopamine production due to neuro-degeneration, which causes disruptions in the brain.[107] Glutamate activity is increased.[108] Serotonin production is severely decreased,[109] as is GABA production.[110] The abnormalities with these chemical signals result in dysfunction such as motor control, tremors, anxiety, depression, and dementia.

In patients with Multiple Sclerosis, an abnormal inflammatory response causes the body's natural inflammation response to attack the neuron. High levels of glutamate also play a role in MS.[111]

Activation of specific endocannabinoid receptors can affect how neurotransmitters behave. In 2006, research in mice suggested activating CB2 receptors may slow the progression of ALS, or Amyotrophic Lateral Sclerosis, also known as Lou Gehrig's Disease.[112]

CBD: Your All-Natural Antioxidant with Known Neuroprotective Qualities

As an antioxidant with known neuroprotective qualities, CBD is thought to provide a plethora of opportunities for people with neurological conditions. The process of oxidation creates free radicals, a contributing factor to Parkinson's disease, and other neurological conditions.

The neuroprotective and antioxidant properties of CBD suppress the release of neurotransmitters, reduce inflammation, neutralize free radicals, and improve motor control and cognitive performance.[113]

CBD & Neurological Disorders: The Research is Compelling

- **Multiple Sclerosis Clinical Trials:** In 2015, researchers from Italy conducted a three-month clinical trial involving 322 patients with Multiple Sclerosis. The results showed that Sativex proved to be effective in improving MS spasticity with few side effects.[114] A previous study, published in 2007 out of London, followed 66 patients over two years, noting a significant improvement in symptoms with few side effects and no tolerance development.

- **ALS Clinical Trial:** A study of 60 ALS patients showed Sativex improved spasticity in terms of severity, as well as frequency. Participants also noted a decrease in pain, better sleep, and improved appetite.[115]

- **Alzheimer's Disease:** In 2016, a promising study of 10 Alzheimer's patients suggested CBD oil is an effective treatment for Alzheimer's disease. Patients reported a significant decrease in symptoms like delusions, agitation or aggression, irritability, apathy, and sleep.[116]

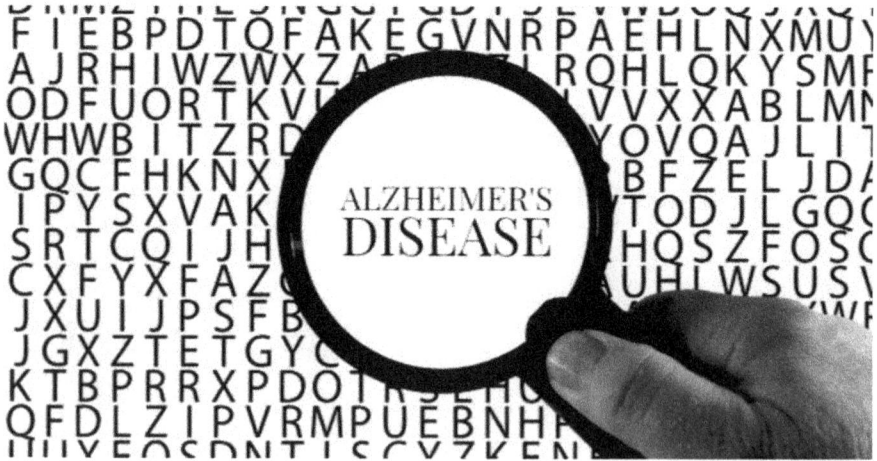

- **General Neurological Research:** A preliminary study from the American Academy of Neurology came out in May of 2019, which stated medical cannabis is safe and effective for a variety of conditions in older people, including ALS, Parkinson's, neuropathy, spinal cord damage, and MS.[117]

What Patients are Saying

Multiple Sclerosis

In an interview,[118] a patient taking sixteen drugs for MS stated, "They gave me a massive cocktail of drugs," he recalls. "Valium for anxiety. Percocet and OxyContin for pain. Ritalin [a stimulant] to keep me from nodding off." He continued, "Steroids.

Antidepressants. Drugs for spasms and digestive issues. And, drugs to treat drug interactions!" The patient successfully eliminated all but one of the 16 drugs with the use of cannabis and recent MRIs show the condition is regressing.

Stroke

A patient that experienced a massive hemorrhagic stroke was left with severe tremors and motor control issues on the left side of his body. He said, "The first time I tried CBD, I immediately felt like I had better sensation, improved control, and almost complete negation of the tremors," he said. "The most incredible thing was that after a few months, I started getting impulses to do things like use my left arm to close the microwave or slide it normally into a shirt sleeve instead of pulling the sleeve onto the left arm with my right hand."[119]

12

AUTOIMMUNE DISORDERS

"I have fibromyalgia pain in my left arm, and the only thing that offers any real relief is cannabis."

— Morgan Freeman, Actor

- Psoriasis
- Celiac Disease
- Lupus
- Fibromyalgia
- Addison's Disease

- Graves' Disease
- Hashimoto's Disease
- Chronic Fatigue Syndrome

According to the American Autoimmune and Related Diseases Association, there are approximately 80-100 autoimmune diseases that affect up to 50 million people.[120] Therefore, it should be no surprise that autoimmune disease is one of the top causes of death in females.

Like other chronic conditions, diagnosis and treatment are challenging. Symptoms of autoimmune disorders can impact multiple organs in the body and require many specialists. Pharmaceutical treatments commonly used to treat these autoimmune disorders can have significant long-term ramifications.

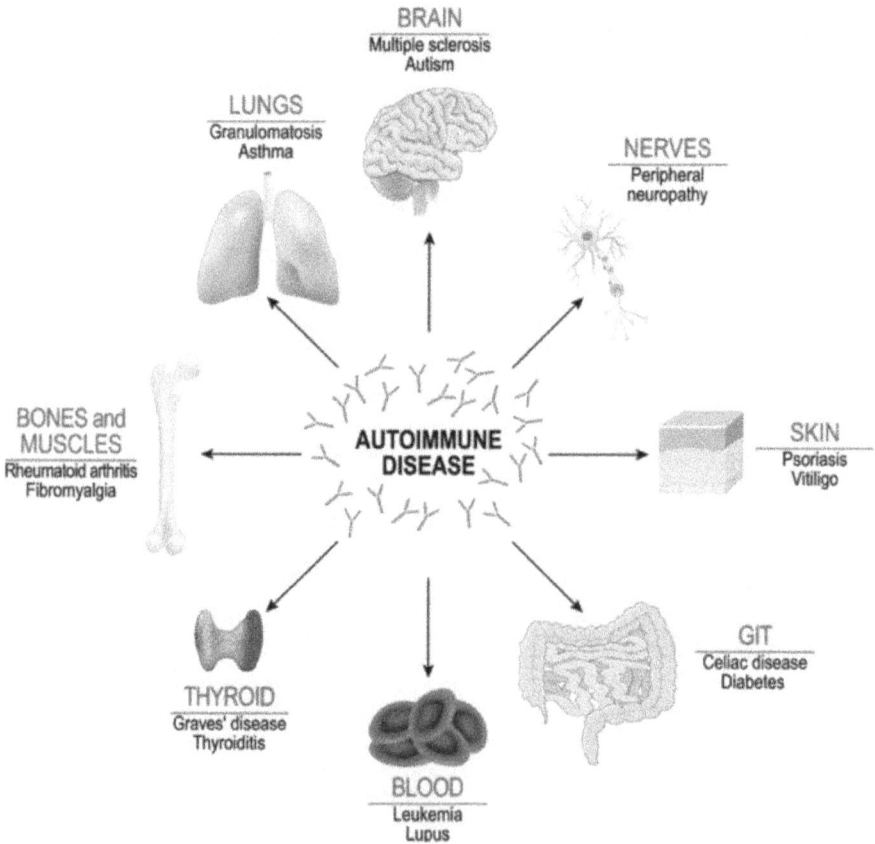

BRAIN
Multiple sclerosis
Autism

LUNGS
Granulomatosis
Asthma

NERVES
Peripheral
neuropathy

BONES and
MUSCLES
Rheumatoid arthritis
Fibromyalgia

**AUTOIMMUNE
DISEASE**

SKIN
Psoriasis
Vitiligo

THYROID
Graves' disease
Thyroiditis

BLOOD
Leukemia
Lupus

GIT
Celiac disease
Diabetes

Autoimmune disorders can be defined as a signaling malfunction that causes the immune system to attack healthy cells within your body. A normally functioning immune system only attacks foreign substances like bacteria, viruses, and cancer. With autoimmune disorders, the immune system may see things like skin, joints, and even organs as a foreign invader. Some autoimmune diseases attack just one area, while others can affect the entire body.

Autoimmune disorders negatively impact us in a multitude of ways. For example, if your immune system attacks your joints, then it may lead to Rheumatoid Arthritis. If your immune system attacks the skin, then the patient is diagnosed with psoriasis. If it attacks the thyroid gland, Hashimoto's is a likely culprit. Diabetes occurs when the immune system takes aim at the pancreas and diseases like Systemic Lupus may manifest in several places such as joints, skin, digestive system, and the brain.[121]

Researchers believe several factors lead to the onset of an autoimmune disease, including genetic predisposition, an imbalance in gut bacteria, and environmental factors.[122] Symptoms of autoimmunity involve fatigue, mild fever, aches and pains, redness, swelling, skin rashes, tingling, and numbness in the limbs as well as an overall lack of health and comfort.

Genetics

Autoimmune
disorder

Environmental
factors

Gut
dysbiosis

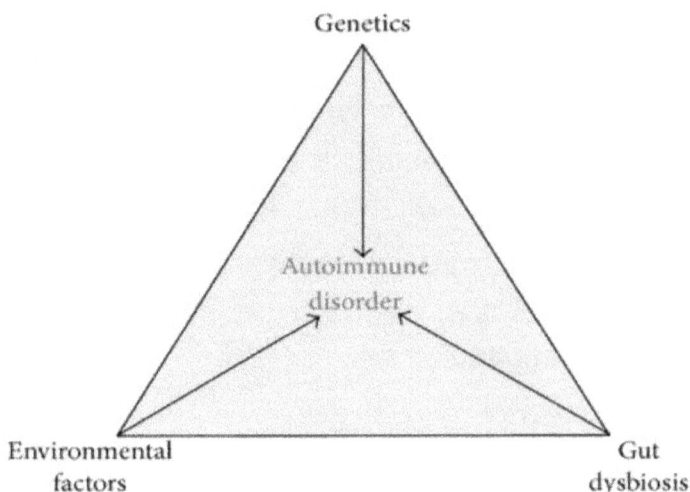

Traditional treatments for autoimmune disorders include anti-inflammatories, such as NSAIDs, immunosuppressant medications, corticosteroids, hormone replacements, and biologic drugs. Besides the known side effects of NSAIDs, immune suppressing agents and pharmaceuticals can increase the risk of disease in patients, and cause nausea, vomiting, trembling, appetite loss, and excessive hair growth. As we discussed, these treatments can become troublesome and often lead to polypharmacy as doctors and patients try to ease adverse side effects.

CBD: Your All-Natural Solution to Autoimmune Disorders

As discussed, the ECS is intertwined with the immune system, and modulating the immune response is part of the process of maintaining homeostasis. Like many other conditions, inflammation is the root of the problem, and reducing inflammation is primary.

CB1 and CB2 receptors are both found on immune cells. In fact, it is estimated that there are between 10-100 times more CB2 receptors than CB1, and since cannabinoids act upon immune cells directly through the CB2 receptors, researchers believe modulating these receptors may have a significant impact on our immune system functions.[123]

Activating CB2 receptors creates an anti-inflammatory effect and has long been a therapeutic target for many types of autoimmune disorders and neurodegenerative diseases. The ability of the ECS to suppress immune activity is generally short-lived, thus not interfering with battling infectious disease when necessary.[124]

CBD & Autoimmune Disorders: The Research is Compelling

Here are several ways cannabinoids may impact autoimmune disorders:

- **Anti-Inflammatory Effects** – CBD can reduce inflammation by slowing the production of pro-inflammatory cells called cytokines. CBD also suppresses T-cell production, which also slows the inflammation response.[125]

- **Gene Expression** – CBD may also increase the expression of genes that control oxidative stress and cell damage, which can contribute to the development of autoimmune issues.[126] In 2013, researchers at the University of South Carolina studied the impact of cannabinoids on microRNAs, molecules that play a role in gene expression. By manipulating these molecules with cannabinoids, scientists observed changes in how the genes were expressed.

- **Immune Modulating** – CBD provides a biphasic response to our endocannabinoid function – a delicate balancing act to keep the systems in our body working regularly. In an article from ProjectCBD,[127] Dr. Mariano Garcia de Palau, a Spanish cannabis clinician, stated, "I believe [cannabis] is immunosuppressive when there is a hyper-immune response, but otherwise it regulates and corrects the immune system. In fact, you could say it functions like the endocannabinoid system, bringing equilibrium to the organism."

What Patients are Saying

Lupus

"...believe me when I tell you that doctors are wrong when they claim there isn't a way to heal? I am reversing my Lupus diagnosis, and I have the lab results to prove it. CBD oil is an effective part of my healing protocol, along with clean, real food, metabolic medicine, and other supplements and treatments."[128]

Grave's Disease

"A year ago, my doctor suggested that I try it because I am so sensitive to a lot of the medications that I need to take for my thyroid and my pain. Most of the medications make me sicker or feel worse, and I certainly don't want to feel worse than I already do... I have a prescription for it and use it legally. Cannabis has saved me from the misery that no one should ever have to go through, be it a Thyroid Storm, RA, Hyperthyroidism, or Hashimoto's."[129]

PART 3

GETTING STARTED WITH CBD

13

HOW TO CHOOSE THE BEST CBD PRODUCTS FOR YOU

"I wanted a healthier, more natural option for pain management, sleep aid, relaxation, and general recovery. CBD has been integral in my training and recovery program."

— Megan Rapinoe, Olympic Soccer Player

One of the benefits of living in today's fast-paced, modern world is the unlimited choices available to us all. CBD supplementation is no exception, with a massive variety of product forms to choose from.

Let's break down the various types of CBD products that are available, explain how they are consumed, their unique bioavailability, and the specific benefits of each product type.

CBD 101: Full Spectrum CBD vs. Broad Spectrum CBD vs. CBD Isolates

As you peruse the various CBD products available, you will frequently see one of three terms on the label: full spectrum, broad spectrum, and isolate. Understanding these terms is critical in choosing the best CBD product for you.

Full Spectrum Hemp Oils

Also called whole-plant extractions, full spectrum extracts are as close to the natural chemical makeup of the original hemp plant as possible.

This means that the test results of the CBD extraction and the raw hemp plant material would be found to contain the same amount of CBD, THC, minor cannabinoids, flavonoids, and terpenes.

Full spectrum hemp derived extracts contain a small amount of THC, which is legally required to be less than 0.3%. **This means that full spectrum CBD is non-psy-**

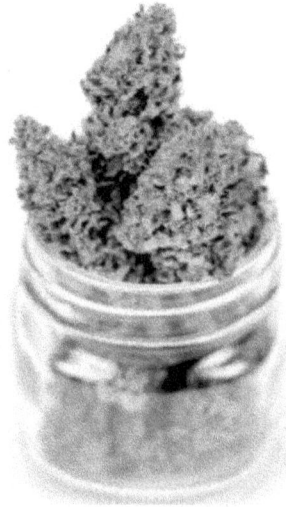

Full-spectrum products contain all the cannabinoids from the original plant & will always contain a small amount of THC. (.3% or less by law)

choactive and won't get you high.

A note about THC: Although a level of .3% will not produce an intoxicating effect, it could, in some cases, cause someone to fail a THC drug screen. Therefore, high-tech lab processes are used to create products that are THC free.

Broad Spectrum Hemp Oils

Many states dictate that CBD products sold over the counter cannot contain any THC at all. To satisfy these requirements, CBD manufacturers use high-tech solutions to remove the THC from the hemp biomass.

Similar to the process of decaffeinating coffee, producers use a process called flash chromatography to remove the THC. After this process, the oil is called broad spectrum CBD. **Both full and broad spectrum CBD products deliver the**

Broad-spectrum products contain all the cannabinoids from the original plant, except for THC.

THC FREE ✓

Isolates only contain one cannabinoid. CBD Isolates are pure cannabidiol (95-99% pure CBD)

benefits of a plethora of active compounds, including several minor cannabinoids, terpenes, and flavonoids.

Researchers have found that when all these compounds are combined together, they work to produce even more significant medical benefits than any single molecule does on its own. As previously discussed, this phenomenon is known as **"The Entourage Effect."**

Cannabinoid Isolates

While full spectrum and broad spectrum oils include a blend of minor cannabinoids, terpenes, and flavonoids, isolates are precisely what their name implies, isolated cannabinoids. CBD isolates are processed to the point where everything, but the CBD, has been stripped away.

The resulting product is a fine, crystalline powder which can then be blended into a wide variety of products, put into capsules, or consumed by vaporizing.

While there are some specific applications for CBD isolates, these products do not provide the consumer with the full therapeutic benefits that full spectrum and broad spectrum CBD offer.

Bioavailability: A Major Factor in Choosing CBD

All of us want to enjoy the maximum amount of benefits that CBD offers to improve our lives. **CBD bioavailability is the**

percentage of CBD that is actually absorbed into your bloodstream. This means that in each and every case, the amount of CBD that is absorbed into your body will be different from the amount listed on the label of the product.

The chart shown below indicates that CBD bioavailability is determined by the type of product form you take.

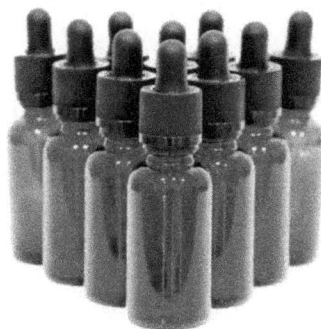

Vaping	Tinctures	Smoking	Edibles	Topicals
50-80%	40-50%	30%	4-20%	5-10%

You Have Endless Ways to Enjoy the Benefits of CBD

CBD Tinctures

Tinctures are one of the most effective and popular ways to take CBD. Tinctures are a liquid cannabinoid extraction, which are consumed by holding the liquid under your tongue, allowing the cannabinoids to be absorbed through the mucous membrane in your mouth rather than inhaled or digested. Tinctures are typically made with alcohol and diluted with water and/or oils. Some manufacturers also add a small amount of flavoring to make the products more palatable.

"As a former professional athlete, CBD is oil for the tin man. I take a CBD tincture daily and use CBD based cream for muscular aches and soreness."

– Marvin Washington, NFL Athlete

A significant benefit of tinctures is that CBD can be consumed without inhalation. While tinctures don't have the same immediate onset as inhalation, it typically only takes about 20 minutes for the patient to start enjoying the benefits. Tinctures are also very convenient, easy to use, and don't emit any odors.

"CBD is popping up everywhere. It's in oils, lotion, toothpaste, bath bombs, shampoo, and even ice cream. It's definitely moved from the experimental fringes to the mainstream."

– Kathy Smith, Fitness, Longevity & Wellness Legend

CBD Edibles and Drinks

Commercially produced CBD edibles and beverages are fast becoming one of the most popular and enjoyable forms of consumption.

A vast array of delicious products, including chocolate bars, baked goods, and hard candies, are available. There is also a large beverage market, including CBD infused water, soda, beer, and tea.

While drinking and eating your CBD is a fun and pleasant way to supplement with cannabinoids, this is not the most efficient way to medicate.

Eating CBD infused food requires digestion, meaning that most of the CBD is broken down by your liver before it is circulated into your bloodstream. This results in a delayed onset time, between 30 minutes and two hours. Additionally, only 4 to 20 percent of the cannabinoids listed on the label are absorbed into your system.

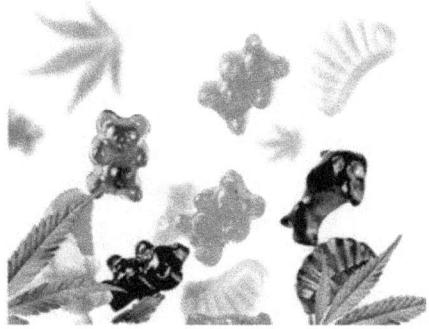

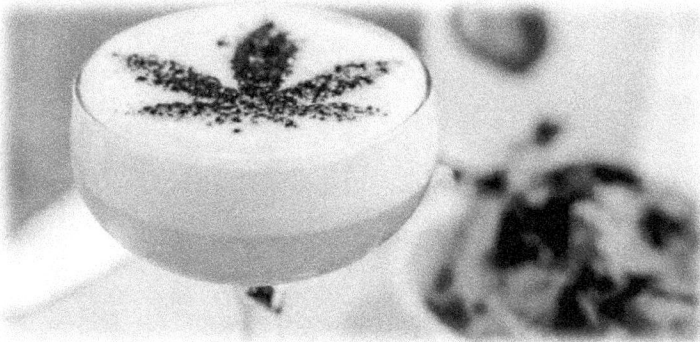

Note: Putting CBD in your coffee, cookies, and candies is all the rage right now. Every corner café from Los Angeles to New York City offers some type of CBD infused goodie on their menu. While this is a great marketing gimmick, it's likely these café treats do not contain enough CBD to provide much of an effect. For best results, stick with commercially produced and tested CBD edibles and beverages that are required to deliver precise dosages and ingredients.

CBD Topicals

CBD based lotions, salves, patches, and bath products are used for localized pain, muscle soreness, arthritis pain, fibromyalgia, and other skin conditions, including burns.

While the obvious benefits of topicals include ease of use and lack of ingestion, there is one significant drawback. Topicals have very low bioavailability, which means just a small fraction of what you apply to your skin actually makes it to your receptors.

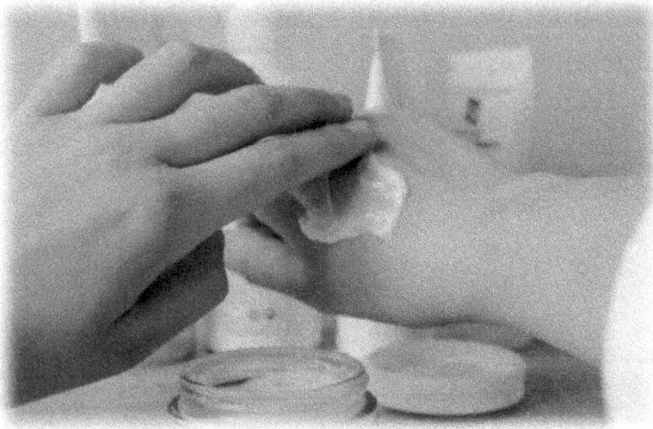

Safety Tip: Always check the ingredients on topical products. Many will contain other beneficial herbs and elements such as lavender, turmeric, menthol, or camphor. Consumers with allergies should be especially diligent in reading labels and monitoring ingredients.

CBD Capsules

CBD capsules are the most familiar and nonthreatening way to begin CBD supplementation. However, just like eating or drinking CBD, tablets are slow to absorb into your bloodstream, and only a fraction of the cannabinoids listed on the label will actually be absorbed into your system.

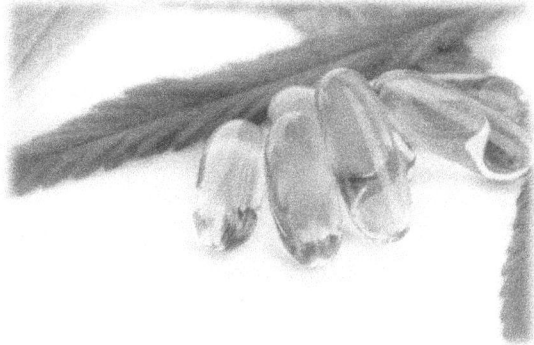

Vaping CBD Oils

If you desire the fast efficacy of inhalation, the new trend of CBD oil vape pens may be the right choice for you. You can purchase a disposable vape pen, or buy pre-filled, disposable cartridges that attach to a battery. Both of these devices heat the CBD oil inside and convert it into a vapor.

Additionally, vaping is convenient, without the mess or odors associated with smoking raw hemp. Vaporizing allows for the quick onset of effects for patients who need an immediate response. However, the benefits will typically wear off relatively quickly, in about an hour or two.

Safety Tip: As you've likely read in recent news, additives in some vape cartridges can be dangerous. In cannabis and hemp, always buy vape cartridges made without any additives or flavorings. Many manufacturers use oils such as MCT oil, propylene glycol (PG) or Polyethylene Glycol (PEG), or Vitamin E to alter the viscosity of the oils. While the FDA considers these additives generally safe for consumption via food products, they have not been tested or proven safe for inhalation.

Smoking CBD

If the multi-billion-dollar tobacco industry has taught us anything, we've learned inhaling smoke has disadvantages. While CBD hemp can be smoked, this isn't the safest and healthiest method of ingestion, especially for patients with lung ailments.

However, inhalation is proven to be the fastest method for the onset of symptom relief. That's because inhaled cannabinoids are immediately introduced into our circulatory system and carried to the appropriate receptors, which is valuable for ailments that require an immediate response such as anxiety. While the benefits from inhaling are experienced quickly, they tend to wear off in an hour or two.

14

5 STEPS TO MINDBLOWING RESULTS

"I had dozens of surgeries and over 20 concussions. I was given opiates, and I'm surprised I'm still alive. CBD is a better alternative. I believe in the healing properties of this plant so much."

— Ryan VanderBussche, NHL Athlete

Congratulations!

You've made it to the end of this book, so now you have all the details and insights on how VALUABLE and LIFE CHANGING CBD supplementation can be.

Deep down inside, you've always known there must be a BETTER SOLUTION out there than the expensive and debilitating lab made pharmaceuticals that are constantly being prescribed to you.

Your intuition is 100% correct!

Clearly, it's time to explore a different path. **At this stage in your life, you deserve to live every single moment, of every single day, exactly as you want.**

CBD can remove the obstacles that stand in your way of enjoying a calm and restful life, free from pain, stress, and anxiety.

After countless hours of research in preparation for this book, here's the best advice I can give you on how to get started with CBD supplementation, right now.

1. Choose a **full spectrum, whole plant CBD!** This means you have selected a product that contains an entire array of minor cannabinoids, terpenes, and flavonoids, so you can enjoy ALL of the potential therapeutic benefits that CBD offers to turn your life around.

2. Make sure your full spectrum, whole plant CBD has less than 0.3% THC so it's **non-psychoactive, and won't get you high!**

3. **Choose CBD products that have been third party tested for potency.** Make sure you receive a Certificate of Analysis (COA) from an unbiased, third party lab that shows your CBD was strictly tested to insure an accurate amount of CBD, as well as a full array of minor cannabinoids, terpenes, and flavonoids.

4. **Choose CBD products that have been third party tested for purity.** The Certificate of Analysis (COA) should also show your CBD has been tested for contaminants including molds, fungus, yeasts, bacteria, and heavy metals.

5. Demand a **Lifetime Guarantee of Quality and Satisfaction!** Never forget, you'll be putting the CBD you choose in and on your body. So, common sense tells us to choose a company that believes in their product as much as you do. Therefore, I advise you to purchase from companies that are willing to guarantee your complete satisfaction.

If for any reason you become dissatisfied with the CBD you choose, you should be entitled to a full and prompt refund, <u>no questions asked!</u>

What to Expect When You Begin CBD Supplementation

When you finally take your first CBD, expect to be BLOWN AWAY!

If you're like most people, after just one dose, you'll have a big "aha" moment.

This will be the moment when a warm calm envelopes you, and your nagging pain, soreness, and worries suddenly begin to melt away.

You'll be amazed at how fast the CBD acts, and you'll be impressed with how good it makes you feel.

Make no mistake about it, this may be the all-natural medical breakthrough that you've been so desperately searching for.

This is finally your chance to wake up from a restful night of sleep with more energy than you had in your youth, and more calm and focus than you could ever expect at this stage of your life.

It's easy to give up on life as we get older. Most people do.

But you're different, because you've read this book. This means you are a naturally curious, open-minded individual willing to consider new ap-

proaches and possibilities.

TODAY is the day to take action. Tomorrow could be too late.

There's no reason to remain stuck in the same old frustrating place you are now.

So, don't wait another moment.

Just this once… do something special for yourself.

Choose CBD!

So, you can start enjoying a much higher quality of life that you always knew was out there for you.

You're going to be OVERJOYED with how things play out!

Yours in Health and Happiness,

Brooke Tilson, MSG

Author, Secret CBD Cures for Seniors

ABOUT THE AUTHORS

Brooke Tilson graduated Summa Cum Laude from the University of Southern California in just three years, and has a Master of Science in Gerontology from USC's Leonard Davis School of Gerontology. Brooke is now dedicating her professional life to greatly improving the health and wellness of Seniors.

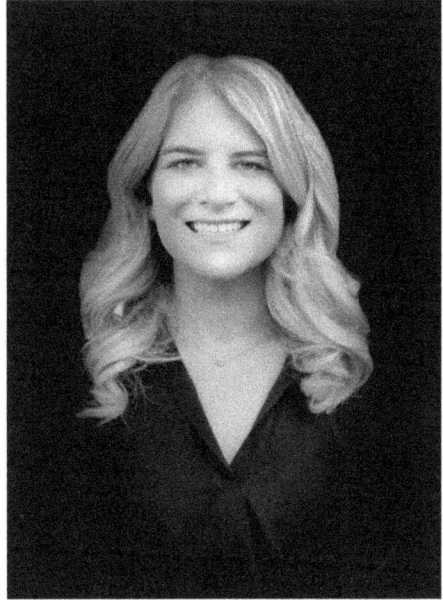

Kristina Etter is the Editorial Director for Cannabis Tech, and is a well-known journalist and public speaker in the cannabis industry. Kristina is committed to combining passion and professionalism to confront and change many of the stigmas attached to the cannabis industry.

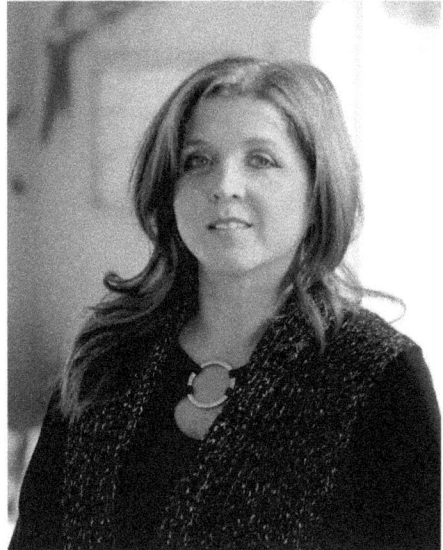

REFERENCES

Chapter 1

1. Preparing for an Aging Population. https://www.aarp.org/livable-communities/about/info-2018/aarp-livable-communities-preparing-for-an-aging-nation.html

2. Ashton Applewhite, TEDtv, *"Let's End Ageism"*, February 11, 2018, https://www.ted.com/talks/ashton_applewhite_let_s_end_ageism

Chapter 3

3. Borchardt, Debra, "Survey: Nearly Half of People Who Use Cannabidiol Products Stop Taking Traditional Medicines," Forbes Magazine, Aug. 2, 2017

4. Nagarkatti, Prakash et al. "Cannabinoids as novel anti-inflammatory drugs." Future medicinal chemistry vol. 1,7 (2009): 1333-49. doi:10.4155/fmc.09.93

5. Xiong W. et al. "Cannabinoids suppress inflammatory and neuropathic pain by targeting α3 glycine receptors." Journal of Experimental Medicine 2012 June 4; 209(6): 1121-34. doi: 10.1084/jem.20120242

6. Booz, George W. "Cannabidiol as an emergent

therapeutic strategy for lessening the impact of inflammation on oxidative stress." Free radical biology & medicine vol. 51,5 (2011): 1054-61. doi:10.1016/j.freeradbiomed.2011.01.007

7. Zanelati, TV, et al, "Antidepressant-like effects of cannabidiol in mice: possible involvement of 5HT1A receptors." British Journal of Pharmacology, 2010 Jan;159(1):122-8. doi: 10.1111/j.1476-5381.2009.00521.x

8. Iffland, Kerstin, and Franjo Grotenhermen. "An Update on Safety and Side Effects of Cannabidiol: A Review of Clinical Data and Relevant Animal Studies." Cannabis and cannabinoid research vol. 2,1 139-154. 1 Jun. 2017, doi:10.1089/can.2016.0034

Chapter 4

9. Ligresti, A., Antitumor activity of plant cannabinoids with emphasis on the effect of cannabidiol on human breast carcinoma," Journal of Pharmacology and Experimental Therapeutics, September 2006, 318(3): 1375-87

10. McAllister, Sean D et al. "The Antitumor Activity of Plant-Derived Non-Psychoactive Cannabinoids." Journal of neuroimmune pharmacology: the official journal of the Society on NeuroImmune Pharmacology vol. 10,2 (2015): 255-67. doi:10.1007/s11481-015-

9608-y

11. Appendino, G. et al, "Antibacterial Cannabinoids from Cannabis sativa: A Structure–Activity Study," J. Nat. Prod.20087181427-1430, August 6, 2008 https://doi.org/10.1021/np8002673, Copyright © 2008 The American Chemical Society and American Society of Pharmacognosy

12. Ruhaak, L. et al, "Evaluation of the Cyclooxygenase Inhibiting Effects of Six Major Cannabinoids Isolated from Cannabis sativa," May 2011, Vol. 34, Issue 5, Pp. 774-778, doi: 10.1248/bpb.34.774

13. Borrelli F. et al, Beneficial effect of the non-psychotropic plant cannabinoid cannabigerol on experimental inflammatory bowel disease," Biochemical Pharmacology, 2013 May; 85(9): 1306-16, doi: 10.1016/j.bcp.2013.01.017

14. Valdeolivas, S., "Neuroprotective properties of cannabigerol in Huntington's disease: studies in R6/2 mice and 3-nitropropionate-lesioned mice," Neuropathics, January 2015, 12(1): 185-99, doi: 10.1007/s13311-014-0304-z

15. Russo, Ethan. (2016). Beyond Cannabis: Plants and the Endocannabinoid System. Trends in Pharmacological Sciences. 37. 10.1016/j.tips.2016.04.005.

16. Goldstein, Bonni, "What is CBG? The 'Stem Cell' of all the Cannabinoids," YouTube, Feb. 12, 2019, https://www.youtube.com/

watch?v=xe7ryxtqhoA&feature=youtu.
be&t=56

17. Pertwee, R., GW Pharmaceuticals, Patent Application #US20100292345A1, https://patents.google.com/patent/US20100292345

18. "Pre-Clinical Trial on Cannabis Active Ingredients Offers Encouraging Results for Insomnia," Sleep Review, February 4, 2019, http://www.sleepreviewmag.com/2019/02/preclinical-trial-cannabis-insomnia/

19. Steep Hill Labs, CBN, https://www.steephill.com/science/cannabinoids

20. "Precision Plant Molecules Introduces the First Commercially Available High Purity Cannabichromene (CBC) Distillate to the Global Canna Marketplace" PR Newswire, August 27, 2019, https://prn.to/30CDTUh

21. Sun, Jidong, PhD, "D-Limonene: Safety and Clinical Applications," Alternative Medicine Review, Vol. 12, No.3, 2007, http://www.altmedrev.com/archive/publications/12/3/259.pdf

22. Russo, E. B. (2011), Taming THC: potential cannabis synergy and phytocannabinoid-terpenoid entourage effects. British Journal of Pharmacology, 163: 1344-1364. doi:10.1111/j.1476-5381.2011.01238.x

23. Chen, W. et al (March 2015), Anti-tumor effect of α-pinene on human hepatoma cell

lines through inducing G2/M cell cycle arrest. Journal of Pharmacological Sciences, 127, 3: 332-338. doi.org/10.1016/j.jphs.2015.01.008

24. Legault, J., Pichette, A. Potentiating effect of beta-caryophyllene on anticancer activity of alpha-humulene, isocaryophyllene and paclitaxel., The Journal of Pharmacy and Pharmacology, 2007 Dec, 59 (12): 1643-7.

25. Mandal, S. et al, Coriander (Coriandrum sativum L.) essential oil: Chemistry and biological activity, Asian Pacific Journal of Tropical Biomedicine, Vol 5:6, 421-428, June 2015

26. Kamatou, G. and Viljoen, A., Linalool – A Review of a Biologically Active Compound of Commercial Importance. Natural Product Communications. 2008, Vol. 3, No. 7 pp 1183-1192. https://journals.sagepub.com/doi/pdf/10.1177/1934578X0800300727

27. Rea, K. et al, Biosynthesis of cannflavins A and B from Cannabis Sativa L. Journal of Phytochemistry. Vol. 164, August 2019, 162-171. doi.org/10.1016/j.phytochem.2019.05.009

Chapter 5

28. Medical students not trained to prescribe medical marijuana: Many states allow medical pot, but few med schools address it, Washington University School of Medicine, September

15, 2017 https://www.sciencedaily.com/releases/2017/09/170915144132.htm

29. Fuss, Johannes et al. "A runner's high depends on cannabinoid receptors in mice." *Proceedings of the National Academy of Sciences of the United States of America* vol. 112,42 (2015): 13105-8. doi:10.1073/pnas.1514996112

30. Zou, Shenglong, and Ujendra Kumar. "Cannabinoid Receptors and the Endocannabinoid System: Signaling and Function in the Central Nervous System." *International journal of molecular sciences* vol. 19,3 833. 13 Mar. 2018, doi:10.3390/ijms19030833

31. Russo, EB. "Clinical endocannabinoid deficiency (CECD): can this concept explain therapeutic benefits of cannabis in migraine, fibromyalgia, irritable bowel syndrome and other treatment-resistant conditions?" *Neuro Endocrinology Letters.* 2004 Feb-Apr;25(1-2):31-9.

32. Russo, Ethan B. "Clinical Endocannabinoid Deficiency Reconsidered: Current Research Supports the Theory in Migraine, Fibromyalgia, Irritable Bowel, and Other Treatment-Resistant Syndromes." Cannabis and cannabinoid research vol. 1,1 154-165. 1 Jul. 2016, doi:10.1089/can.2016.0009

33. Pacher, Pál, and George Kunos. "Modulating the endocannabinoid system in human health and disease--successes and failures." The FEBS journal vol. 280,9 (2013): 1918-43. doi:10.1111/

febs.12260

Chapter 6

34. Charlesworth, Christina J et al. "Polypharmacy Among Adults Aged 65 Years and Older in the United States: 1988-2010." *The journals of gerontology. Series A, Biological sciences and medical sciences* vol. 70,8 (2015): 989-95. doi:10.1093/gerona/glv013

35. David, Edgar G., VP of Corporate Affairs, Eli Lilly & Company, 1984 US House of Representative, https://www.ncbi.nlm.nih.gov/pmc/articles/PMC2690298/figure/fig01/

36. Think You're Seeing More Drug Ads on TV? You Are, And Here's Why. New York Times, December 24, 2017. https://www.nytimes.com/2017/12/24/business/media/prescription-drugs-advertising-tv.html

37. Al Ameri MN, Makramalla E, Albur U, Kumar A, Rao P (2014) Prevalence of Poly-pharmacy in the Elderly: Implications of Age, Gender, Co-morbidities and Drug Interactions. SOJ Pharm Pharm Sci, 1(3), 1-7. DOI: http://dx.doi.org/10.15226/2374-6866/1/3/00115

38. "The other big drug problem: Older people taking too many pills," The Washington Post, December 9, 2017, https://www.washingtonpost.com/national/health-science/the-other-big-drug-problem-older-people-

taking-too-many-pills/2017/12/08/3cea5ca2-
c30a-11e7-afe9-4f60b5a6c4a0_story.html

Chapter 7

39. Mental Illness Statistics. National Institute of
     Mental Health. February 2019. https://www.
     nimh.nih.gov/health/statistics/mental-illness.
     shtml#part_154785

40. Walker, Elizabeth Reisinger et al. "Insurance
     status, use of mental health services, and unmet
     need for mental health care in the United
     States." *Psychiatric services (Washington, D.C.)*
     vol. 66,6 (2015): 578-84. doi:10.1176/appi.
     ps.201400248

41. Mental Health and Chronic Diseases. CDC.
     National Healthy Worksite. Issue Brief No.
     2, October 2012. https://www.cdc.gov/
     workplacehealthpromotion/tools-resources/
     pdfs/issue-brief-no-2-mental-health-and-
     chronic-disease.pdf

42. Parks, J., et al. National Association of State
     Mental Health Program Directors Council.
     (2006). Morbidity and Mortality in People
     with Serious Mental Illness. http://www.
     nasmhpd.org/docs/publications/MDCdocs/
     Mortality%20and%20Morbidity%20Final%20
     Report%208.18.08.pdf

43. Project CBD, How CBD Works. https://www.

projectcbd.org/how-cbd-works

44. Eisenstein, Michael. The reality behind cannabidiol's medical hype. Nature. August 28, 2019. https://www.nature.com/articles/d41586-019-02524-5

45. Mental Health Daily, High Dopamine Levels: Symptoms & Adverse Reactions. http://mentalhealthdaily.com/2015/04/01/high-dopamine-levels-symptoms-adverse-reactions/

46. Reflected on the Mind, The Effects of Glutamate in the Treatment of Anxiety Disorders.http://reflectd.co/2013/04/03/anxiety-medication-the-effects-of-glutamate-in-the-treatment-of-anxiety-disorders/

47. Daniel C. Matthews, et al. July 9, 2012.The National Center for Biotechnology Information, Targeting the Glutamatergic System to Treat Major Depressive Disorder. https://www.ncbi.nlm.nih.gov/pmc/articles/PMC3439647

48. Project CBD, How CBD Works. https://www.projectcbd.org/how-cbd-works

49. José Alexandre de Souza Crippa, et al. October 29, 2003. Nature.com, Neuro-pyschopharmacology Journal, Effects of Cannabidiol (CBD) on Regional Cerebral Blood Flow. http://www.nature.com/npp/journal/v29/n2/full/1300340a.html

50. Poddar MK and Dewey WL. July 1980. The National Center for Biotechnology Information,

Effects of cannabinoids on catecholamine uptake and release in hypothalamic and striatal synaptosomes. https://www.ncbi.nlm.nih.gov/pubmed/7391971

51. Project CBD, How CBD Works. https://www.projectcbd.org/how-cbd-works

52. Bergamaschi MM, et al. February 9, 2011. The National Center for Biotechnology Information, Cannabidiol reduces the anxiety induced by simulated public speaking in treatment-naïve social phobia patients. https://www.ncbi.nlm.nih.gov/pubmed/21307846

53. José Alexandre S Crippa, et al. September 9, 2010. Journal of Psychopharmacology, Neural basis of anxiolytic effects of cannabidiol (CBD) in generalized social anxiety disorder: a preliminary report. http://journals.sagepub.com/doi/full/10.1177/0269881110379283

54. Kopf, Dan & Avins, Jenni, "New data show Americans are turning to CBD as a cure-all for the modern condition," Quartz, April 15th, 2019, https://qz.com/1590765/survey-shows-americans-use-cbd-to-treat-anxiety-and-stress/

55. Dolgoff, S. Does CBD Oil Work for Anxiety? I Tried it to Find Out. Good Housekeeping. July 8, 2019. https://www.goodhousekeeping.com/

health/wellness/a27197249/what-is-cbd-oil/

Chapter 8

56. Dahlhamer J, Lucas J, Zelaya, C, et al. Prevalence of Chronic Pain and High-Impact Chronic Pain Among Adults — United States, 2016. MMWR Morb Mortal Wkly Rep 2018;67:1001–1006 DOI: http://dx.doi.org/10.15585/mmwr. mm6736a2

57. Guy GP Jr., Zhang K, Bohm MK, et al. Vital Signs: Changes in Opioid Prescribing in the United States, 2006–2015. MMWR Morb Mortal Wkly Rep 2017;66:697–704. DOI: http://dx.doi.org/10.15585/mmwr.mm6626a4

58. Mojtabai, R. National trends in long-term use of prescription opioids. *Pharmacoepidemiol Drug Saf.* 2018; 27:526– 534. https://doi.org/10.1002/pds.4278

59. The Effects of Opioid Use, American Addiction Centers, https://drugabuse.com/opiates/effects-of-use/

60. Tarone RE, Blot WJ, McLaughlin JK. Nonselective nonaspirin nonsteroidal anti-inflammatory drugs and gastrointestinal bleeding: relative and absolute risk estimates from recent epidemiologic studies. Am J Ther. 2004;11(1):17-25.

61. Singh G, Triadafilopoulos G. Epidemiology of NSAID induced gastrointestinal complications.

J Rheumatol. 1999;26(Suppl 56):18-24.

62. Boehnke, Kevin F., Qualifying Conditions of Medical Cannabis License Holders in The United States. Health Affairs 2019 38:2, 295-302

63. Russo, Ethan B. "Cannabinoids in the management of difficult to treat pain." Therapeutics and clinical risk management vol. 4,1 (2008): 245-59. doi:10.2147/tcrm.s1928

64. Nagarkatti, Prakash et al. "Cannabinoids as novel anti-inflammatory drugs." *Future medicinal chemistry* vol. 1,7 (2009): 1333-49. doi:10.4155/fmc.09.93

65. Pertwee, R. G. (2008). The diverse CB1 and CB2 receptor pharmacology of three plant cannabinoids: Δ9-tetrahydrocannabinol, cannabidiol and Δ9-tetrahydrocannabivarin. British Journal of Pharmacology, 153(2), 199–215. http://doi.org/10.1038/sj.bjp.0707442

66. Carrier, E. J., Auchampach, J. A., & Hillard, C. J. (2006). Inhibition of an equilibrative nucleoside transporter by cannabidiol: A mechanism of cannabinoid immunosuppression. Proceedings of the National Academy of Sciences of the United States of America, 103(20), 7895–7900. http://doi.org/10.1073/pnas.0511232103

67. FA, Iannotti & Hill, Charlotte & A, Leo & Alhusaini, Ahlam & Soubrane, Camille & Mazzarella, Enrico & Russo, Emilio & Whalley, Benjamin & Marzo V, Di & Stephens,

Gary. (2014). The non-psychotropic plant cannabinoids, cannabidivarin (CBDV) and cannabidiol (CBD), activate and desensitize transient receptor potential vanilloid 1 (TRPV1) channels in vitro: potential for the treatment of neuronal hyperexcitability.. ACS Chemical Neuroscience. .

68. Marks, D. M., Shah, M. J., Patkar, A. A., Masand, P. S., Park, G.-Y., & Pae, C.-U. (2009). Serotonin-Norepinephrine Reuptake Inhibitors for Pain Control: Premise and Promise. Current Neuropharmacology, 7(4), 331–336. http://doi.org/10.2174/157015909790031201

69. O'Sullivan, S. E. (2016). An update on PPAR activation by cannabinoids. British Journal of Pharmacology, 173(12), 1899–1910. http://doi.org/10.1111/bph.13497

70. Kathmann M, Flau K, Redmer A, Trankle C, Schlicker E. Cannabidiol is an allosteric modulator at mu- and delta-opioid receptors. Naunyn Schmiedebergs Arch Pharmacol. 2006;372(5):354–61.

71. Elmes, M. W., Kaczocha, M., Berger, W. T., Leung, K., Ralph, B. P., Wang, L., ... Deutsch, D. G. (2015). Fatty Acid-binding Proteins (FABPs) Are Intracellular Carriers for Δ9-Tetrahydrocannabinol (THC) and Cannabidiol (CBD). The Journal of Biological Chemistry, 290(14), 8711–8721. http://doi.org/10.1074/

jbc.M114.618447

72. Nurmikko, Turo et al. (2007). Nurmikko TJ, Serpell MG, Hoggart B, Toomey PJ, Morlion BJ, Haines D. Sativex successfully treats neuropathic pain characterised by allodynia: a randomised, double-blind, placebo-controlled clinical trial. Pain 133: 210-220. Pain. 133. 210-20. 10.1016/j.pain.2007.08.028.

73. R Johnson, Jeremy, et al (2009). Multicenter, Double-Blind, Randomized, Placebo-Controlled, Parallel-Group Study of the Efficacy, Safety, and Tolerability of THC:CBD Extract and THC Extract in Patients with Intractable Cancer-Related Pain. Journal of pain and symptom management. 39. 167-79. 10.1016/j.jpainsymman.2009.06.008.

74. Blake DR, Robson P, Ho M, Jubb RW, et al. Preliminary assessment of the efficacy, tolerability and safety of a cannabis-based medicine (Sativex) in the treatment of pain caused by rheumatoid arthritis. Rheumatology (Oxford) 2006;45:50–2.

75. Wilsey, B., et al (2016). An Exploratory Human Laboratory Experiment Evaluating Vaporized Cannabis in the Treatment of Neuropathic Pain from Spinal Cord Injury and Disease. The Journal of Pain: Official Journal of the American Pain Society, 17(9), 982–1000. http://doi.org/10.1016/j.jpain.2016.05.010

76. H Andreae, Michael, et al. (2015). Inhaled

cannabis for chronic neuropathic pain: an individual patient data meta-analysis. The journal of pain: official journal of the American Pain Society. 16. 10.1016/j.jpain.2015.07.009.

77. N Rhyne, Danielle, et al (2016). Effects of Medical Marijuana on Migraine Headache Frequency in an Adult Population. Pharmacotherapy. 36. 505-510. 10.1002/phar.1673.

78. Fiz, J., Durán, M., Capellà, D., Carbonell, J., & Farré, M. (2011). Cannabis Use in Patients with Fibromyalgia: Effect on Symptoms Relief and Health-Related Quality of Life. PLoS ONE, 6(4), e18440. doi.org/10.1371/journal.pone.0018440

Chapter 9

79. Gill, L., Can CBD Help You Sleep?, Consumer Reports, February 6, 2019, https://www.consumerreports.org/cbd/can-cbd-help-you-sleep/

80. McCabe, A., The Disturbing Side Effects of Ambien, No. 1 Prescription Sleep Aid, Huffington Post, February 23, 2016 https://www.huffpost.com/entry/ambien-side-effect-sleepwalking-sleep-aid_n_4589743

81. Frank A.J.L. Scheer, Hungry for Sleep: A Role for Endocannabinoids?, Sleep, Volume 39, Issue 3, March 2016, Pages 495–496, https://

doi.org/10.5665/sleep.5510

82. Lights Out for Insomnia: New Kanabo Research Study Offers Encouraging Results, PRNewswire: https://www.prnewswire.com/ il/news-releases/lights-out-for-insomnia-new-kanabo-research-study-offers-encouraging-results-300785925.html

83. Russo, Ethan B., Guy, Geoffrey W. and Robson, Philip J. (2007), Cannabis, Pain, and Sleep: Lessons from Therapeutic Clinical Trials of Sativex®, a Cannabis-Based Medicine. Chemistry & Biodiversity, 4: 1729–1743. doi:10.1002/cbdv.200790150

84. Chagas, Marcos Hortes N., et al. "Effects of Acute Systemic Administration of Cannabidiol on Sleep-Wake Cycle in Rats." Journal of Psychopharmacology, vol. 27, no. 3, Mar. 2013, pp. 312–316, doi:10.1177/0269881112474524.82 Shannon, Scott et al. "Cannabidiol in Anxiety and Sleep: A Large Case Series." *The Permanente journal* vol. 23 (2019): 18-041. doi:10.7812/ TPP/18-041

85. Shannon, Scott et al. "Cannabidiol in Anxiety and Sleep: A Large Case Series." The Permanente journal vol. 23 (2019): 18-041. doi:10.7812/TPP/18-041

Chapter 10

86. Cancer Statistics. National Institute for Health.

National Cancer Institute. https://www.cancer.gov/about-cancer/understanding/statistics

87. Side Effects of Cancer Treatment. National Cancer Institute. https://www.cancer.gov/about-cancer/treatment/side-effects

88. Josée Guindon and Andrea G Hohmann. August 2011. The National Center for Biotechnology Information, The endocannabinoid system and cancer: therapeutic implication. https://www.ncbi.nlm.nih.gov/pmc/articles/PMC3165955/

89. Blanca Herrera, et al. August 2006. The National Center for Biotechnology Information, The CB2 cannabinoid receptor signals apoptosis via ceramide-dependent activation of the mitochondrial intrinsic pathway. https://www.ncbi.nlm.nih.gov/pubmed/16624285

90. M Solinas, et al. November 2012.The National Center for Biotechnology Information, Cannabidiol inhibits angiogenesis by multiple mechanisms. https://www.ncbi.nlm.nih.gov/pmc/articles/PMC3504989/

91. Clarice MacGarvey. March 31, 2016. Discover CBD, Can CBD Oil Help Minimize Oxidative Stress? https://discovercbd.com/blogs/cbd-news/99087878-can-cbd-oil-help-minimize-oxidative-stress

92. RP Rocconi, et al. April 2008. The National Center for Biotechnology Information, Lipoxygenase pathway receptor expression in ovarian cancer. https://www.ncbi.nlm.nih.gov/

pubmed/18421027

93. Paola Massi, et al. February 2013. The National Center for Biotechnology Information, Cannabidiol as potential anticancer drug. https://www.ncbi.nlm.nih.gov/pmc/articles/ PMC3579246/

94. M Mimeault, et al. June 15, 2003. The National Center for Biotechnology Information, Anti-proliferative and apoptotic effects of anandamide in human prostatic cancer cell lines: implication of epidermal growth factor receptor down-regulation and ceramide production. https:// www.ncbi.nlm.nih.gov/pubmed/12746841

95. LJ Crofford. July 1997. The National Center for Biotechnology Information, COX-1 and COX-2 tissue expression: implications and predictions. https://www.ncbi.nlm.nih.gov/ pubmed/9249646

96. Luciano De Petrocellis, et al. July 7, 1998. The National Center for Biotechnology Information, The endogenous cannabinoid anandamide inhibits human breast cancer cell proliferation. https://www.ncbi.nlm.nih.gov/pmc/articles/ PMC20983/

97. Matthew W. Elmes, et al. April 3, 2015. The National Center for Biotechnology Information, Fatty Acid Binding Proteins (FABPs) are Intracellular Carriers for Δ9-Tetrahydrocannabinol (THC) and Cannabidiol (CBD). https://www.ncbi.nlm.nih.gov/pmc/

articles/PMC4423662/

98. P Massi, et al. March 2004. The National Center for Biotechnology Information, Antitumor effects of cannabidiol, a nonpsychoactive cannabinoid, on human glioma cell lines. https://www.ncbi.nlm.nih.gov/pubmed/14617682

99. Sean D. McAllister, et al. November 2007. American Association for Cancer Research, Cannabidiol as a novel inhibitor of Id-1 gene expression in aggressive breast cancer cells. http://mct.aacrjournals.org/content/6/11/2921

100. Sindiswa T. Lukhele and Lesetja R. Motadi. September 1, 2016. The National Center for Biotechnology Information, Cannabidiol rather than Cannabis sativa extracts inhibit cell growth and induce apoptosis in cervical cancer cells. https://www.ncbi.nlm.nih.gov/pmc/articles/PMC5009497/

101. B Romano, et al. April 15, 2014. The National Center for Biotechnology Information, Inhibition of colon carcinogenesis by a standardized Cannabis sativa extract with high content of cannabidiol. https://www.ncbi.nlm.nih.gov/pubmed/24373545

102. A. E. Munson, L. S. Harris, M. A. Friedman, W. L. Dewey, R. A. Carchman, Antineoplastic Activity of Cannabinoids, JNCI: Journal of the National Cancer Institute, Volume 55, Issue 3, September 1975, Pages 597–602, https://doi.

org/10.1093/jnci/55.3.597

103. Scott, K. A., Dalgleish, A. G., Liu, W. M."Anticancer effects of phytocannabinoids used with chemotherapy in leukemia cells can be improved by altering the sequence of their administration". International Journal of Oncology 51.1 (2017): 369-377.

104. Preet, Anju et al. "Cannabinoid receptors, CB1 and CB2, as novel targets for inhibition of non-small cell lung cancer growth and metastasis." Cancer prevention research (Philadelphia, Pa.) vol. 4,1 (2011): 65-75. doi:10.1158/1940-6207. CAPR-10-0181

105. Manju Sharma, et al. July 2014. Scientific research Publishing SCIRP, In Vitro Anticancer Activity of Plant-Derived Cannabidiol on Prostate Cancer Cell Lines. http://www.scirp.org/journal/PaperInformation. aspx?PaperID=47691#.U8FwiKiAQUF

Chapter 11

106. Gooch, C. L., Pracht, E. and Borenstein, A. R. (2017), The burden of neurological disease in the United States: A summary report and call to action. Ann Neurol., 81: 479-484. doi:10.1002/ana.24897

107. Galvan, A., & Wichmann, T. (2008). Pathophysiology of Parkinsonism. Clinical Neurophysiology: Official Journal of

the International Federation of Clinical Neurophysiology, 119(7), 1459–1474 http://doi.org/10.1016/j.clinph.2008.03.017

108. Johnson, K. A., Conn, P. J., & Niswender, C. M. (2009). Glutamate receptors as therapeutic targets for Parkinson's disease. CNS & Neurological Disorders Drug Targets, 8(6), 475–491.

109. Marios Politis, Flavia Niccolini, Serotonin in Parkinson's disease, In Behavioural Brain Research, Volume 277, 2015, Pages 136-145, ISSN 0166-4328, https://doi.org/10.1016/j.bbr.2014.07.037. http://www.sciencedirect.com/science/article/pii/S0166432814004860

110. Błaszczyk, J. W. (2016). Parkinson's Disease and Neurodegeneration: GABA-Collapse Hypothesis. Frontiers in Neuroscience, 10, 269. http://doi.org/10.3389/fnins.2016.00269

111. IR Stojanovic, et al. March 15, 2014. The National Center for Biotechnology Information, The role of glutamate and its receptors in multiple sclerosis. https://www.ncbi.nlm.nih.gov/pubmed/24633998

112. Kathline Kim, Dan H. Moore, Alexandros Makriyannis, Mary E. Abood, AM1241, a cannabinoid CB2 receptor selective compound, delays disease progression in a mouse model of amyotrophic lateral sclerosis, In European Journal of Pharmacology, Volume 542, Issues 1–3, 2006, Pages 100-105, ISSN 0014-2999,

https://doi.org/10.1016/j.ejphar.2006.05.025. http://www.sciencedirect.com/science/article/pii/S0014299906005103.

113. Hampson, A. J., Grimaldi, M., Axelrod, J., & Wink, D. (1998). Cannabidiol and (−)Δ9-tetrahydrocannabinol are neuroprotective antioxidants. Proceedings of the National Academy of Sciences of the United States of America, 95(14), 8268–8273.

114. M. Trojano and C. Vila. November 17, 2015. The National Center for Biotechnology Information, Effectiveness and Tolerability of THC/CBD Oromucosal Spray for Multiple Sclerosis Spasticity in Italy: First Data from a Large Observational Study. https://www.ncbi.nlm.nih.gov/pubmed/26571097

115. Nilo Riva, MD, PhD. (2015). A Fase II, Randomized, Double-Blind, Placebo-Controlled, Multicentre Study for the Safety and Efficacy on Spasticity Symptoms of a Cannabis Sativa Extract in Motor Neuron Disease Patients. Retrieved from https://clinicaltrials.gov/ct2/show/record/NCT01776970.

116. Shelef A, et al. 2016. The National Center for Biotechnology Information, Safety and Efficacy of Medical Cannabis Oil for Behavioral and Psychological Symptoms of Dementia: An-Open Label, Add-On, Pilot Study. https://www.ncbi.nlm.nih.gov/pubmed/26757043

117. Press Release. Could Medical Marijuana Help

Grandma and Grandpa with their Ailments? American Academy of Neurology. February 28, 2019. https://www.aan.com/PressRoom/Home/PressRelease/2698

118. Kossen, J. Cannabis and Multiple Sclerosis Treatment. Leafly.com 2016 https://www.leafly.com/news/health/medical-cannabis-multiple-sclerosis-treatment

119. Dodgson, L., Baby boomers were once demonized for using marijuana, but now they're swearing by it as a miracle cure. Insider, May 31, 2019, https://www.insider.com/baby-boomers-using-marijuana-for-mental-health-pain-ageing-problem-2019-5

Chapter 12

120. American Autoimmune Related Diseases Association, Autoimmune Disease Statistics. Last Updated 2018 https://www.aarda.org/news-information/statistics/#1488234386508-a9560084-9b69

121. National Institute of Environmental Health Sciences. https://www.niehs.nih.gov/health/topics/conditions/autoimmune/index.cfm

122. Campbell, Andrew. Autoimmunity and the Gut. Autoimmune Diseases. May 2014 doi: 10.1155/2014/152428

123. Turcotte, C. et al, The CB2 receptor and its role as a regulator of inflammation. Cellular and

Molecular Life Sciences. 2016; 73(23): 4449–4470. doi: 10.1007/s00018-016-2300-4

124. Rupal Pandey, Khalida Mousawy, Mitzi Nagarkatti, and Prakash Nagarkatti. Endocannabinoids and immune regulation. Pharmacol Res. 2009 Aug; 60(2): 85–92, doi: 10.1016/j.phrs.2009.03.019

125. Kozela, E, et all. "Pathways and gene networks mediating the regulatory effects of cannabidiol, a nonpsychoactive cannabinoid, in autoimmune T cells" J Neuroinflammation. 2016

126. Hegde, Venkatesh L et al. "Distinct microRNA expression profile and targeted biological pathways in functional myeloid-derived suppressor cells induced by Δ9-tetrahydrocannabinol in vivo: regulation of CCAAT/enhancer-binding protein α by microRNA-690." The Journal of biological chemistry vol. 288,52 (2013): 36810-26. doi:10.1074/jbc.M113.503037

127. Biles, M., *Cannabis and the Immune System: A complex balancing act*. Project CBD. https://www.projectcbd.org/science/cannabis-and-immune-system

128. How CBD Oil Permanently Changed My Autoimmune Condition. https://www.thefix.com/how-cbd-oil-permanently-changed-my-autoimmune-condition

129. Bacom-Stone, Jackie. "How Cannabis Has Helped My Thyroid Disease. Dec. 2014.

Thyroid Nation. https://thyroidnation.com/cannabis-helped-thyroid-disease/

INDEX

A

B

C

Cancer

Brain Cancer 87
Breast Cancer 23, 87, 88, 144, 145
Cancer Pain
  See *Chronic Pain Conditions*
Cervical Cancer 88
Colon Cancer 81
Leukemia 81, 89
Lung Cancer 81, 89
Pancreatic Cancer 81
Prostate Cancer 89

Cannabinoids

Cannabichromene 26
Cannabidiol 11
Cannabigerol 23
Cannabinol 25
THC 11, 13, 16, 22, 25, 68, 77, 89, 110, 111

Cardiovascular System 38, 39, 54

CBD Products 109–118

CBD Beverages 115
CBD Capsules 117
CBD Edibles 115, 116
CBD Flower 118
CBD Tinctures 113
CBD Topicals 116
CBD Vapes xviii–153, 117

CED

  See *Clinical Endocannabinoid Deficiency*

Certificate of Analysis 121

Chronic Pain Conditions 63–71

www.ingramcontent.com/pod-product-compliance
Lightning Source LLC
Chambersburg PA
CBHW022108280326
41933CB00007B/303